Management of Cataracts and Glaucoma

Edited by

Anne Louise Coleman, MD PhD
Professor of Ophthalmology and Epidemiology
Director of Center for Eye Epidemiology
Frances and Ray Stark Chair in Ophthalmology
Jules Stein Eye Institute
University of California
Los Angeles, CA, USA

John C. Morrison, MD
Professor of Ophthalmology
Director of Glaucoma Service
Casey Eye Institute
Oregon Health and Science University
Portland, OR, USA

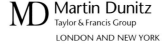
MD Martin Dunitz
Taylor & Francis Group
LONDON AND NEW YORK

© 2005 Taylor & Francis, an imprint of the Taylor & Francis Group

First published in the United Kingdom in 2005
by Taylor & Francis, an imprint of the Taylor & Francis Group, 2 Park
Square, Milton Park, Abingdon, Oxfordshire, OX14 4RN

Tel.:   +44 (0) 20 7017 6000
Fax.:   +44 (0) 20 7017 6699
E-mail: info@dunitz.co.uk
Website: http://www.dunitz.co.uk

Although every effort has been made to ensure that all owners of
copyright material have been acknowledged in this publication,
we would be glad to acknowledge in subsequent reprints or editions
any omissions brought to our attention.

A CIP record for this book is available from the British Library.

Library of Congress Cataloging-in-Publication Data

Data available on application
ISBN 1 84184 271 0

Distributed in North and South America by
Taylor & Francis
2000 NW Corporate Blvd
Boca Raton, FL 33431, USA
Within Continental USA
Tel.: 800 272 7737; Fax.: 800 374 3401
Outside Continental USA
Tel.: 561 994 0555; Fax.: 561 361 6018
E-mail: orders@crcpress.com

Distributed in the rest of the world by
Thomson Publishing Services
Cheriton House
North Way
Andover, Hampshire SP10 5BE, UK
Tel.: +44 (0)1264 332424
E-mail: salesorder.tandf@thomsonpublishingservices.co.uk

Composition by J&L Composition, Filey, North Yorkshire

Printed and bound in Spain by Grafos SA

Contents

List of Contributors

George Baerveldt MBChb FCS
Irving H Leopold Professor and Chair
Department of Ophthalmology
UCI Medical Center
Irvine, CA 92697, USA

Michelle C Banks MD
Assistant Professor of Ophthalmology
Jules Stein Eye Institute
UCLA School of Medicine
100 Stein Plaza
Los Angeles CA 90095–7004
USA

Keith Barton MD MRCP FRCS
Consultant Ophthalmologist
Moorfields Eye Hospital
162 City Road
London EC1V 2PD
UK

Joseph Caprioli MD
Professor of Ophthalmology
Chief, Glaucoma Division
Jules Stein Eye Institute
UCLA School of Medicine
100 Stein Plaza
Los Angeles CA 90095–7004
USA

Fathi El-Sayyad FRCS FCOphth
El-Maghraby Eye Hospital
Jeddah
Saudi Arabia

Howard V Gimbel MD MPH FACS FRCSC
Medical Director
Gimbel Eye Centre
4935 40th Avenue NW, Suite 450
Calgary, AB T3A 2N1
Canada

Richard A Hill MD
Associate Professor of Ophthalmology
University of California, Irvine
25 Zola Court
Irvine CA 92612–4061
USA

Kyoko Ishida MD PhD
Research Fellow
University of Tennessee
Memphis, TN, USA

John G Ladas MD PhD FACS
Assistant Professor of Ophthalmology
Wilmer Eye Institute, Maumenee 327
Johns Hopkins University
600 North Wolfe Street
Baltimore MD 21287–9238
USA

Jean E Keamy MD MBA
Clinical Instructor of Ophthalmology
Tufts School of Medicine
136 Harrison Avenue
Boston, MA 02111, USA

André Mermoud MD

Jules Gonin Eye Hospital

Avenue de France 15

CH-1004 Lausanne

Switzerland

Richard Mills MD MPH

Clinical Professor of Ophthalmology

University of Washington

1221 Madison St, Suite 1124

Seattle, WA 98104, USA

Paul Palmberg MD PhD

Bascom Palmer Eye Institute

University of Miami

School of Medicine

900 NW 17th Street

Miami FL 33136

USA

Paul E Pentheroudakis

Department of Anesthesia

UCLA

Los Angeles, CA 90054, USA

Sheila P Sanders, MD

Department of Ophthalmology and Visual Sciences

University of Kentucky

140 South Limestone E308

Lexington KY 40536

USA

Tarek Shaarawy MD

Chef, Unité du Glaucome

Clinique d'opthamologie

Hôpitaux Universitaires de Genève

22 rue Alcide Jentzer

1211 Genève 14

Switzerland

Walter J Stark MD

Professor of Ophthalmology

Wilmer Eye Institute, Maumenee 327

Johns Hopkins University

600 North Wolfe Street

Baltimore MD 21287–9238

USA

Brandon L Villarreal MD

Assistant Professor of Anesthesiology

Department of Anesthesiology

The David Geffen School of Medicine at UCLA

The Center for the Health Sciences

Los Angeles, California 90054, USA

Preface

Treatment of patients with both cataracts and glaucoma requires diagnostic skill and keen clinical judgment. Ophthalmologists treating these patients must decide whether to recommend surgery and, if so, they must determine the timing of surgery, the type of procedure to perform, and details of the surgical approach. Recent experience suggests a trend toward greater use of combined cataract and glaucoma procedures in older individuals in the USA. In the US Medicare population aged 65 years or older, there were approximately 51 900 combined cataract and trabeculectomy procedures performed between 1996 and 1999 compared with 28 080 trabeculectomies only.

Despite this popularity, there has been only limited evidence-based demonstration of the benefit of combined cataract and glaucoma procedures. In 2002, Dr Henry Jampel and coauthors reported that from 1964 to July 2000 there were 36 randomized controlled trials on combined surgery (Ophthalmology 2002; 109: 1892–901). In their review of the literature, they found 'excellent' support for the conclusion that postoperative intraocular pressure (IOP) tends to be lower 24 hours after a combined cataract and glaucoma procedure than 24 hours after a cataract extraction alone. They also reported 'fair' evidence that the use of mitomycin C produced slightly lower IOPs than surgery without antimetabolites, that two-site surgery provided slightly lower IOPs than one-site surgery, and that 5-fluorouracil did not improve IOP reduction.

It is clear that clinical trials have a limited ability to determine the relative value of all of the nuances among surgical techniques. For this reason, ophthalmic surgery will remain an art that depends heavily on the skill and judgment of the surgeon. In this book, we have asked highly regarded, expert glaucoma surgeons to present their strategic thinking and to share pearls of wisdom with ophthalmic surgeons who face the challenge of treating patients with both cataracts and glaucoma.

In the first chapter, Drs Brandon Villarreal and Paul Pentheroudakis, anesthesiologists at the David Geffen School of Medicine at UCLA, discuss the philosophy and challenges of ophthalmic anesthesia in routine, pediatric, and sick individuals. Drs John Ladas and Walter Stark of the Wilmer Eye Institute at Johns Hopkins Medical School discuss surgical management of patients when the surgeon favors cataract extraction either by itself or to be followed by glaucoma surgery. Subsequent chapters consider trabeculectomy only (described by Dr Keith Barton of Moorefields Hospital, London, UK), drainage device implantation (presented by Drs Richard Hill and George Baerveldt of the University of California in Irvine), and nonpenetrating filtering surgery (described by Drs Tarek Shaarawy and André Mermoud of the University of Lausanne, Switzerland). Drs Paul Palmberg and Kyoko Ishida of the Bascom Palmer Eye Institute at the University of Miami present their results with one-site combined cataract and phacoemulsification procedures. Drs Joseph Caprioli and Michelle Banks at the Jules Stein Eye Institute, David Geffen School of Medicine, UCLA discuss issues and surgical approaches for the two-site combined procedure. Dr Sheila Sanders of the University of Kentucky and Dr Richard Mills of the University of Washington in Seattle tackle the difficult issue of a combined cataract extraction and drainage device implantation, Drs Shaarawy, Fathi El-Sayyad, and Mermoud present their surgical approach for a combined phacoemulsification and nonpenetrating filtering surgery, and Drs Howard Gimbel and Jean Keamy at the Gimbel Eye Centre in Calgary, Canada, present surgical approaches for phacoemulsification combined with either endocyclophotocoagulation or trabeculotomy.

In every chapter, the authors present insights and approaches gleaned from years of surgical experience. Clearly, given the nature of surgical medicine and the emerging state of the art, there may be other surgeons with different opinions and approaches. In addition, the majority of surgeries discussed in this book have not been evaluated in randomized clinical trials, so the evidence for their safety and efficacy may be weak. Despite this, we are convinced that the discussions presented here will provide an important framework for fostering exchange of information and cross-fertilization of ideas, so important to this discipline of ophthalmic surgery, where detail matters greatly. This is why we have pursued the writing of this book.

Anne Louise Coleman and John C. Morrison

Acknowledgments

We would like to acknowledge all of our contributors. This book would not exist without their willingness to share their considerable expertise and to devote many hours to preparing their chapters. In addition, we would like to acknowledge Cynthia Reyes, who has devoted numerous hours to the compilation and editing of this book during her undergraduate studies at UCLA.

Dedication

We dedicate this book to our families and patients.

1. Anesthesia for cataract and glaucoma surgery

Brandon L Villarreal and Paul E Pentheroudakis

INTRODUCTION

The anesthesiologist possesses the knowledge and technical skills to provide the ophthalmologist with a safe and comfortably anesthetized patient, while monitoring the patient's cardiorespiratory status during intraocular ophthalmic procedures. With an anesthesiologist, the ophthalmologist is allowed the opportunity to focus solely on their operative technique and ensure a successful operative outcome. The operative eye is akinetic, the intraocular pressure is controlled, and the oculocardiac reflex is either avoided or easily managed by the observant anesthesiologist.

Anesthesiologists provide the ophthalmologist with a safe operative environment by focusing on the patient's immediate cardiorespiratory status, and by continually anticipating and addressing anesthetically those cardiac and respiratory perturbations that may potentially disrupt the ophthalmologist's quiet operative field; this includes excessive intraocular hypertension (acute glaucoma), cardiac arrhythmias, pulmonary hypoxia and hypercarbia (elevated blood carbon dioxide concentration), patient agitation leading to uncontrollable movement, and neurologic disorientation from drug interactions or intra- or extracranial illnesses during monitored anesthesia care (MAC).

Patients undergoing phacoemulsification with intraocular lens implants are often elderly with underlying chronically stable cardiorespiratory disease. Elderly patients with new-onset, unstable cardiorespiratory conditions, such as myocardial ischemia, bradyarrhythmias, tachyarrhythmias, prolonged QT-syndrome, and excessive hypertension (diastolic blood pressure exceeding 110 mmHg), are not candidates for an elective operative procedure, unless the ophthalmologist informs the anesthesiologist of the urgent need to proceed. In such circumstances, the operative procedure will proceed safely while the anaesthetist monitors the patient's cardiorespiratory status with the possible use of an arterial line, Swan–Ganz catheter, or transesophageal probe (TEE).

Infantile glaucoma, congenital glaucoma, and congenital cataracts occur in the very young, whereas acquired cataracts secondary to diabetes or advanced age often appear in older individuals. Very young and elderly patients present the anesthesiologist with unique anesthetic challenges which, when professionally managed, allow the anesthesiologist to successfully provide the ophthalmologist with a quiet operative field and the patient with a safe operating environment.

This chapter focuses on the anesthetic challenges that anesthesiologists address during intraocular cataract and glaucoma surgery.

OVERVIEW

Anesthesiologists provide an invaluable service not only to the ophthalmologist, but also to the patient, their family, and the institution where the operation is taking place. Patients do not want to experience pain nor do they wish to experience anxiety, and most expect complete amnesia of all surgical events, even while receiving MAC. Thus the anesthesiologist's capacity to exhibit humility, warmth, and professional confidence is tested. Communicating in a clear and concise manner is often all that is necessary to allay the patient's anxiety and fear. A sedative-hypnotic is often administered to the anxious patient to help chemically alleviate their anxiety.

Anesthesiologists work in collaboration with nurses and supporting personnel to effectively ensure a smooth transition from operative case to operative case; when an operating room is managed efficiently and is functioning smoothly, the ophthalmologist is able to control and focus their efforts on

1

the surgery. Thus, each patient who enters an operating room is cared for by a team of professionals that anticipates and responds to the tasks necessary in providing a safe and efficient operating experience for the patient and their family.

The anesthesiologist who is cognizant of the ophthalmologist's personal style, anesthetic expectations, and operative behavior will be able to provide a better and safer anesthetic to the patient. Moreover, clear, supportive and constructive communication between the anesthesiologist and the operative surgeon protects the patient under stressful and highly unpredictable anesthetic and operative circumstances.

BASICS OF ANESTHESIA FOR THE PRACTICING OPHTHALMOLOGIST

Anesthesiologists practicing ophthalmologic anesthesia are capable of delivering either general anesthesia or MAC. Under general anesthesia, the airway is supported by the anesthesiologist and the patient is completely anesthetized. During MAC, the patient is comfortably sedated and completely indifferent to the environment, breathing spontaneously without the support of the anesthesiologist and responsive to commands. During the performance of a retrobulbar or peribulbar block, the patient should remain completely motionless (except for breathing) and the eye rendered akinetic. This form of MAC is referred to as 'conscious sedation,' as opposed to 'deep sedation' (in which case the patient may in fact be unconscious) or 'general anesthesia.' The unconscious patient is apneic, at risk for hypoxia and hypercarbia, incapable of protecting his or her airway in the event of vomiting, and at risk for sustained and uncontrollable movements. If the latter do occur during the performance of a retrobulbar block, the surgeon may misdirect the needle and damage the patient's eye.

'Conscious sedation' is provided by the intravenous administration of either remifentanil 0.25–1.5 microgram/kg, alfentanil 10–30 microgram/kg, propofol 10–40 mg, or methohexital (Brevital) 20 to 40 mg. All these medications, par-

ticularly remifentanil, produce 'intense analgesia', so that during a retrobulbar or peribulbar block, the patient remains responsive to commands, is comfortably sedated, and is breathing without any pain; in fact, the patient may appear awake.

All practicing anesthesiologists prefer to have access to the patient's airway while delivering MAC or general anesthesia. However, during an ophthalmologic procedure, the patient's airway must necessarily remain out of the anesthesiologist's physical reach, being extremely close to the operative site and draped with a sterile covering. Therefore, the anesthesiologist needs to be highly observant while continually assessing the patient for unpredictable circumstances that may prevent the patient from breathing effectively. In such circumstances, the anesthesiologist should have at hand numerous airway devices in many different sizes to help ensure patency of the patient's airway. Examples include the oral RAE endotracheal tube, laryngeal mask airway, nasal airway, oral airway, and fiberoptic intubating scope (Figure 1.1). Anesthesiologists also employ a multitude of monitoring devices with built-in alarms that alert them as to the adequacy and effectiveness of oxygenation and ventilation. For example, anesthesia machines possess an alarm that sounds when positive pressure is no longer being administered to the patient via the anesthetic circuit and endotracheal tube, signifying a 'circuit disconnect' (Figure 1.2).

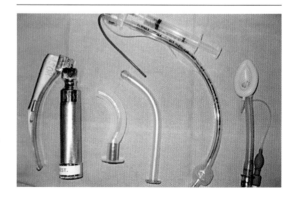

Fig. 1.1 Devices used by anesthesiologists. From left to right: laryngoscope handle attached to laryngoscope blade, various size endotracheal tubes, and a laryngeal mask airway.

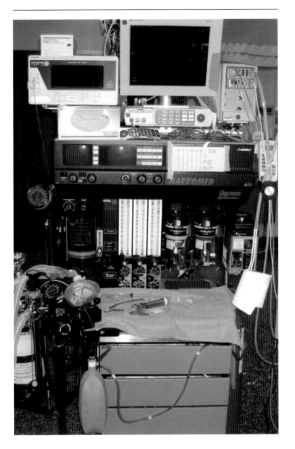

Fig. 1.2 An anesthesia machine with a monitor.

and pulmonary capillary wedge pressure to help differentiate a failing left ventricle from worsening pulmonary hypertension. The SWAN will also measure cardiac output and mixed venous oxygen saturation, which all together help in guiding vasoactive and inotropic drug therapy in addition to intravenous fluid and blood product administration. TEE provides the most sensitive and earliest marker of ischemia and is excellent in assessing adequacy of preload. However, considerable expertise is required to perform and interpret the TEE exam. All these monitoring devices, used together, help to ensure that a consistent and adequate supply of oxygen is delivered to metabolizing tissues; this is especially important for the patient with cardiopulmonary disease.

PREOPERATIVE EVALUATION OF INFANTS AND YOUNG CHILDREN

The infant or child with a congenital cataract will be followed by the ophthalmologist to assess both cataract progression and the development of amblyopia. Often the child will undergo an exam under anesthesia (EUA), which poses a unique challenge to the anesthesiologist. These patients may also have concurrent illnesses and, if needed, the anesthesiologist should be clinically prepared to adjust the anesthetic plan to meet the unique requirements of the patient's underlying illness.

Ex-premies (preterm infants born before 37 weeks gestation) and infants with mental retardation or developmental delay are exquisitely sensitive to sedative-hypnotics (midazolam, propofol, barbiturates), narcotics (fentanyl, alfentanil, remifentanil), and all inhalational agents (sevoflurane, desflurane, isoflurane). Given that most anesthetics decrease myocardial conduction and myocardial contractility, infants under anesthesia are at an increased risk for cardiorespiratory arrest should bradycardia occur.

It requires skill and experience to effectively induce anesthesia using bag–mask ventilation in an infant. In comparison to adults, infants and small children possess a proportionately large occiput

Additionally, oxygen saturation is monitored with a pulse oximeter and carbon dioxide elimination is measured with a capnograph. Multichannel electrocardiogram capability is employed to assess for cardiac ischemia, myocardial infarction, and arrhythmias. An automated blood pressure cuff may be used to noninvasively measure blood pressure every 3–5 minutes. Although most cataract and glaucoma surgeries are elective, urgent surgery in an unstable patient is occasionally indicated. In these cases, more invasive blood pressure monitoring involves placement of an arterial line, which is used when beat-to-beat blood pressure changes or frequent blood draws (electrolytes, blood gases) are required. A Swan Ganz catheter (SWAN) may be used to measure both pulmonary artery pressure and tongue, a long epiglottis, and laryngeal structures that are small and anteriorly displaced (glottic opening located at C4 versus C5–6 in adults). Thus, direct laryngoscopy may be extremely difficult for the inexperienced operator. In addition, infants are prone to laryngospasm, which could quickly lead to hypoxia and hypercarbia, exacerbated by a highly active metabolic rate compared with that of adults. Any time laryngospasm occurs, bronchospasm may also occur. The bronchospasm may be so severe that it may be impossible to ventilate the infant's lungs, in which case hypoxia and hypercarbia rapidly ensue.

In infants, it may be quite difficult to place an intravenous line; thus, the anesthesiologist will need to perform tasks quickly while constantly anticipating those anesthetic circumstances that may compromise the cardiorespiratory reserve of the infant. Before starting the case, the anesthesiologist needs to have in place those tools and medications necessary to establish and maintain cardiorespiratory integrity. These include varying sizes of oral airways and laryngeal mask airways to help deliver oxygen. In addition, atropine and epinephrine need to be readily available, for intravenous and/or endotracheal tube delivery, in order to support the infant's cardiac output.

The infant with congenital glaucoma typically has a diagnosis of primary congenital glaucoma, although a small percentage will have Sturge–Weber syndrome with cerebral calcifications and a seizure disorder. An infant typically presents to the operating room for an EUA; pertinent medical history is obtained, the airway is thoroughly examined, and the patient is assessed for any recent upper respiratory infections (URIs). Patients with a recent URI (within 30 days), have an increased risk of developing laryngospasm and bronchospasm. In these cases it then should be determined, with the ophthalmologist, as to the necessity of proceeding with an EUA. All inhalational agents are active bronchodilators that may improve oxygenation and ventilation (carbon dioxide elimination) during the operative procedure. However, by far the greatest risk occurs during both the induction and the emergence of anesthesia, when the patient may experience both laryngospasm and bronchospasm due to airway instrumentation.

Immediately following mask-induction with sevoflurane, corneal diameters, axial lengths by ultrasound, and refractive error can be measured. Retinoscopy, gonioscopy, ophthalmoscopy, and fundus photography may be performed to evaluate the extent and progression of the patient's glaucoma. All of these measurements and examinations require an *akinetic* eye. Bear in mind that infants may present to the operating room having already received topical glaucoma therapy such as 0.25%–0.50% timolol or betaxolol, topical carbonic anhydrase inhibitors (5–10 mg/kg per oral acetazolamide), and topical sympathomimetics or parasympathomimetics. Timolol and betaxolol are associated with pulmonary bronchoconstriction, particularly in the asthmatic child or infant with a history of bronchopulmonary dysplasia, bronchiolitis, or a recent upper respiratory infection.

Infants may routinely undergo repeated examinations under anesthesia to assess the progression of their glaucoma. It is therefore imperative that, during the initial visit, the anesthesiologist instills both trust and confidence in the infant's parents, since the infant will most likely be returning for multiple EUAs and surgical procedures.

PREOPERATIVE EVALUATION OF THE ELDERLY PATIENT

The elderly patient undergoing glaucoma and cataract surgery, needs to first be evaluated for systemic illnesses, with direct emphasis on their cardiac status, respiratory reserve, hepatic and renal function, and neurological status. It is important to assess the patient's mental capacity and ability to communicate and understand commands, as well as to determine if tremors are present, because the patient must remain immobile during the placement of a retrobulbar block and the surgery itself. Hepatic and renal functions are important for their capacity to metabolize and eliminate the anesthetics that are employed during the administration of general anesthesia and MAC.

Adult patients, particularly those who are older, need to be evaluated for the presence of an arrhythmia and/or ischemic heart disease. Patients with angina should be assessed to determine whether the angina is stable (unchanging chest pain pattern) or unstable (chest pain with worsening pattern or chest pain present at rest). A patient with stable angina can safely proceed with elective surgery assuming proper medical management and appropriate intraoperative monitoring. Unstable angina requires further cardiac evaluation prior to undergoing elective surgery. Patients with diabetes need their cardiac status evaluated prior to surgery because they may have compensated congestive heart failure (CHF) secondary to systolic and/or diastolic dysfunction. The importance of evaluating patients with angina and CHF, especially with a history of a myocardial infarction, is to assess the left ventricular function and the amount of myocardium at risk for ischemia.

The risk of an intraoperative stroke is higher in patients with new-onset atrial fibrillation. Additionally, adult patients with prolonged QT intervals may develop sustained ventricular tachydysrhythmias or bradydysrhythmias with heart block, and might therefore have in place a functioning pacemaker or automatic implantable cardiac defibrillator (AICD). There are more than 1500 models of pacemakers, all programmed with a myriad of functions. The basic purpose of a pacemaker is to permanently pace the atrium and/or the ventricle. Since pacemakers have so many idiosyncratic responses to a variety of intraoperative stimuli ('Bovie' electrocautery, mechanical ventilation), pacemaker magnets should be made available to treat any intraoperative pacemaker emergency. However, pacemakers are programmed to switch into any of a variety of sensing and pacing modes when in contact with a magnet. Therefore, prior to any elective surgery, it is imperative that the pacemaker manufacturer is contacted to determine magnet response and that the pacemaker is 'interrogated' by a programmer (cardiologist, electrophysiologist) to reveal current settings. Automatic implantable cardiac defibrillators (AICDs) are able to recognize hemodynamically significant ventricular tachycardia or ventricular fibrillation and treat them by either pacing or delivering a shock. Therefore, it is absolutely imperative that the AICD is interrogated and disabled prior to surgery in order to prevent the delivery of inappropriate shocks to the patient. Of course a backup cardioverter/defibrillator should be readily available should a malignant ventricular tachydysrhythmia develop intraoperatively.

Adult patients undergoing MAC or general anesthesia should have sufficient respiratory reserve sufficient to sustain their capacity to both oxygenate and ventilate their lungs. The degree of pulmonary reserve an individual has depends on many factors, including the presence of pulmonary disease, history of smoking, obesity, advanced age, and the degree of surgical stress. A thorough medical history, physical examination, chest radiograph, arterial blood gas results, and/or pulmonary function tests all help the anesthesiologist estimate the patient's respiratory reserve. In addition, changing mental status, worsening hypercarbia and/or hypoxia, dyspnea, and tachypnea can help to predict impending ventilatory failure in those with severe respiratory disease. Any pulmonary dysfunction must be medically optimized prior to surgery.

Patients with poorly controlled diabetes should have their blood glucose concentration closely monitored during surgery. Hypoglycemia (blood glucose <50 mg/dl) should be avoided because, if left untreated, it can lead to coma. Because hyperglycemia (blood glucose >250 mg/dl) may result in an increased risk for infection, impaired wound healing, and worsening neurologic outcome following cerebral ischemia, it is recommended that patients have blood glucose levels <250 mg/dl.

Patients taking oral steroids should be evaluated for hyperglycemia, systemic hypertension, fluid retention and metabolic perturbations, particularly acidosis and hyperkalemia.

OPHTHALMOLOGIC AND ANESTHETIC DRUG INTERACTIONS

All sedative-hypnotics, anxiolytics and analgesics employed by anesthesiologists reduce the heart's ability to conduct an action potential along its conduction pathways. Thus, when an intraocular parasympathomimetic, such as acetylcholine, which may also reduce the heart's ability to conduct, is used to promote miosis following lens extraction, patients may develop hypotension and bradycardia. Anesthesiologists can give 0.2–0.4 mg of intravenous (IV) atropine or 5–10 mg of IV ephedrine to reverse the systemic effects of intraocular acetylcholine.

The parasympathomimetic, echothiophate, is a long-acting anticholinesterase which may be used to reduce intraocular pressure. Echothiophate prolongs the action of the short-acting depolarizing muscle relaxant, succinylcholine, by reducing the activity of pseudocholinesterase (which metabolizes succinylcholine). Because of the prolonged muscle relaxant effects, patients using echothiophate preoperatively will most likely need postoperative mechanical ventilation to maintain oxygenation and ventilation if succinylcholine was used intraoperatively. Therefore, nondepolarizing muscle relaxants like rocuronium and vecuronium, whose metabolism is unaffected by echothiophate, can be used when muscle relaxation is necessary.

Intracameral epinephrine is used intraoperatively to pharmacologically dilate pupils during cataract surgery. The absorption of epinephrine from the anterior chamber is minimal, because the iris contains a rich supply of adrenergic receptors that tightly bind epinephrine, preventing its absorption into the blood stream. However, when absorbed systemically, epinephrine is associated with agitation, systemic hypertension, angina pectoris, tachycardia, and ventricular dysrhythmias. If systemic hypertension does occur intraoperatively, the anesthesiologist may start the patient on an intravenous infusion of nitroglycerin or sodium nitroprusside to protect the myocardium from ischemia and prevent the patient from having a cerebral stroke.

Cyclopentolate 2%, a cycloplegic agent, is associated with central nervous system disorientation and overt psychotic reactions. Because disoriented patients may move uncontrollably, become apneic, and/or vomit and aspirate intragastric contents, they should be intubated immediately to provide airway protection and to maintain oxygenation and ventilation.

Phenylephrine 10%, a mydriatic agent occasionally used preoperatively to dilate the pupils for cataract surgery, is associated with systemic hypertension and tremulousness. Systemic absorption may be reduced with the more commonly used 2.5% solution. When a patient with ischemic heart disease systemically absorbs phenylephrine, they are at an increased risk of myocardial ischemia or infarction, tachyarrhythmias, and cardiogenic shock.

In patients with very elevated eye pressures, the anesthesiologist can be asked to administer, either preoperatively or intraoperatively, intravenous mannitol or acetazolamide. Mannitol (1.5–2 g/kg) is always administered slowly over 60 minutes. When administered quickly, it may induce congestive heart failure, myocardial ischemia, pulmonary edema and hypertension followed by hypotension. In addition, it may cause renal failure in patients with poor renal reserve. Mannitol is also associated with hypokalemia and sodium imbalances in patients with normal renal function. Acetazolamide, a carbonic anhydrase inhibitor, should be administered judiciously in patients with renal dysfunction. Systemic administration may lead to hyponatremia and metabolic acidosis. In patients with hepatic dysfunction, acetazolamide is metabolized slowly so the risk for side effects is increased.

Calcium channel blockers and/or β-blockers are also used to treat glaucoma. Because of their effect on the heart's conduction system, electrocardiograms should be assessed for bradyarrhythmia, atrioventricular conduction delays, ventricular escape beats, signs of ischemia, and ventricular fibrillation or tachycardia.

ANESTHETIC CONSIDERATIONS: MONITORED ANESTHESIA CARE

MAC encompasses a spectrum of anesthesia, including anxiolysis, conscious sedation, deep sedation, and general anesthesia. Many of the operative procedures employed for cataracts and glaucoma can be performed with topical anesthetic eye drops, intracameral lidocaine, conscious sedation, or general anesthesia. Most of these operative procedures are performed using conscious sedation with retrobulbar or peribulbar blocks (lidocaine and/or marcaine).

The ideal anesthetic for conscious sedation is one that not only provides intense analgesia during the retrobulbar block but is also rapidly eliminated, thereby avoiding patient disorientation so that they remain comfortable, immobile, responsive to commands, and able to protect their airway.

Intravenous alfentanil (20 microgram/kg) or remifentanil (0.2–1.5 microgram/kg) are extremely short-acting narcotic agents that provide intense analgesia. The patient is able to be indifferent to the sensation and pain of the injection, yet maintain consciousness and the ability to follow commands. Methohexital (Brevital), and other short-acting barbiturates, cause central nervous system depression that may result in unconsciousness. However, unlike narcotics, barbiturates do not provide analgesia and in low doses may even cause disorientation and agitation. Patients given barbiturates are, therefore, more likely to move in response to a painful stimulus.

Midazolam (Versed; 0.5–1.0 mg IV), a benzodiazepine, and propofol (10–75 mg IV), may also be employed to provide anxiolysis and conscious sedation. Benzodiazepines bind with specific receptors in the central nervous system and enhance the inhibitory effects of various neurotransmitters. For example, midazolam facilitates γ-aminobutyric acid (GABA) receptor binding, causing an increase in the transmembrane conduction of chloride ions, thereby inhibiting neuronal function. Propofol may also involve facilitation of GABA transmission.

Patients will rarely require a jaw lift maneuver to open an obstructed airway following the administration of alfentanil, remifentanil, midazolam, or propofol alone. However, simultaneous administration of at least two of these drugs can synergistically enhance their cardiovascular and respiratory depressant effects. Thus, unless the anesthesiologist is aware of the need to temporarily perform a jaw lift maneuver, these patients may have a greater probability of becoming apneic and suffering hemodynamic compromise, and possibly requiring resuscitative maneuvers.

ANESTHETIC CONSIDERATIONS: ORBITAL, FACIAL, AND PERIBULBAR BLOCKS

A retrobulbar block is performed to provide akinesis of the globe (Figure 1.3). With the eye in a neutral position or the patient looking upward and inward, a 25-gauge, 31-mm retrobulbar needle is passed into the muscle cone of the globe, from the inferotemporal quadrant of the orbit, and the needle is directed upward and nasally towards the orbital apex to decrease the possibility of the needle coming into contact with the optic nerve and central retinal artery. If the local anesthetic is mistakenly injected into the meningeal sheath of the optic nerve, the central retinal artery or into the brain stem, 50% of patients will have respiratory impairment for as long as 7 minutes, which requires airway resuscitative measures. Patients may also manifest cardiovascular collapse.

The most common complication of a retrobulbar block is a retrobulbar hemorrhage. Whenever a hemorrhage develops within the orbit, the patient is at risk for the oculocardiac reflex being stimulated, particularly if the optic nerve is not completely anesthetized. Special retrobulbar needles, which have a blunt tip, reduce the chance of perforating retrobulbar vessels and the optic nerve sheath.

Peribulbar blocks appear to be safer than retrobulbar blocks because there have been no reported cases of central nervous system infiltration or

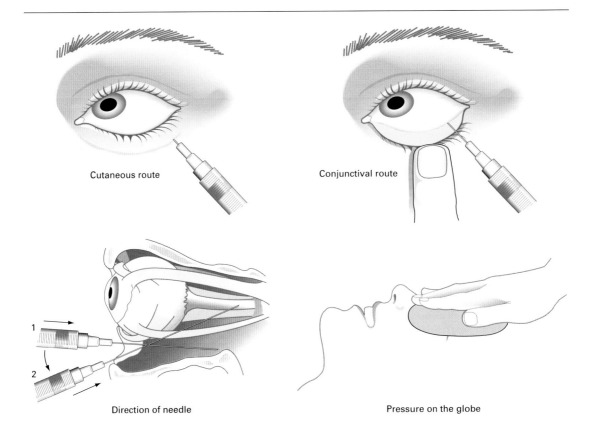

Cutaneous route

Conjunctival route

Direction of needle

Pressure on the globe

Fig. 1.3 Diagram illustrating retrobulbar block.

retrobulbar hemorrhage related to this technique. A peribulbar block involves two injections placed inferotemporally and superonasally in the orbit (Figure 1.4). The injections use twice the volume of local anesthetic and have a slower onset of action compared with retrobulbar blocks. When performing peritubular and retrotubular blocks, orienting the needle bevel towards the globe (Figure 1.4) will decrease the chances of globe perforation.

Akinesis of the eyelids may be obtained by blocking branches of the facial nerve that supply the orbicularis oculi muscle. Facial nerve blocks may be used as an adjunct to retrobulbar or peribulbar blocks. There are multiple techniques for blocking the facial nerve. From proximal to distal, the blocks include the O'Brien, Atkinson, and van Lint (Figure 1.5). Subcutaneous hemorrhage is the major complication of these blocks. Another technique, the Nadbath–Rehman method, blocks the facial nerve at the outlet of the stylomastoid foramen beneath the external auditory canal. Due to this block's proximity to the vagus and glosspharyngeal nerves, it is associated with hoarseness, dysphagia, central agitation, respiratory compromise, and laryngospasm of the vocal cords causing respiratory distress, making it a dangerous block to perform.

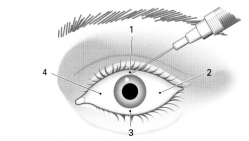

Subconjunctival infiltration anesthesia

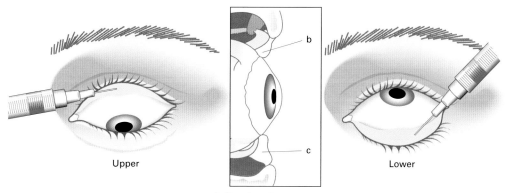

Upper

Infiltration of the cul-de-sac

Lower

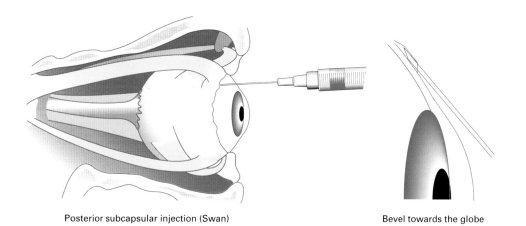

Posterior subcapsular injection (Swan)

Bevel towards the globe

Fig. 1.4 Diagram illustrating peribulbar block.

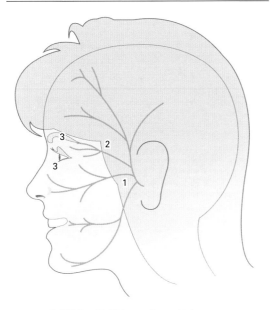

1. O'Brien **2**. Atkinson **3**. van LInt

Fig. 1.5 Diagram illustrating facial nerve blocks.

ANESTHETIC CONSIDERATIONS: OCULOCARDIAC REFLEX

The oculocardiac reflex, or trigeminal–vagal reflex, is a well-described reflex arc. The afferent pathway of this reflex arc is mediated via the trigeminal nerve (CN III) and the efferent limb is via the vagus nerve. The oculocardiac reflex can be initiated by pressure on the eyeball, traction on the extraocular muscles, or during injection of a retrobulbar block. Electrocardiographically it is manifested as cardiac dysrhythmias, including sinus bradycardia, junctional rhythm, or sinus arrest. Although a small percentage of patients may actually have sinus arrest, typically one will see a sinus pause followed by sinus rhythm. This reflex occurs approximately 17–80% of the time in patients undergoing ocular manipulation.

Prophylactic atropine, epinephrine, or norepinephrine are not reliable in preventing the oculocardiac reflex. When the oculocardiac reflex occurs, the ophthalmologist should be immediately notified and instructed to cease further surgical stimulation until the heart rate returns toward baseline. Bradycardia usually resolves after 10 seconds. After repeated stimulation, the reflex arc will usually fatigue, and there will be progressively fewer episodes of bradycardia. If the inciting stimulus (i.e. pulling on the extraocular muscles) has been removed and a prolonged episode of sinus bradycardia or sinus arrest persists, then 0.2–0.4 mg of atropine may be administered intravenously to help stimulate the heart.

ANESTHETIC CONSIDERATIONS: PREVENTION OF RAPID INCREASE IN INTRAOCULAR PRESSURE AND GAGGING

Direct laryngoscopy and endotracheal intubation are highly stimulating to the patient's airway, potentially causing the release of catecholamines, which may cause hypertension, tachycardia and an increase in orbital venous pressure and intraocular pressure. In adults, this stress response to laryngoscopy and intubation can be reduced with either 1.0 mg/kg of IV lidocaine, 100–300 microgram of IV nitroglycerin, 10–20 microgram of IV nitroprusside, or 10–40 mg of IV esmolol delivered just prior to and during intubation.

Because infants and young children might have separation anxiety as well as varying degrees of apprehension related to the proposed procedure, they can be given 0.5–1.2 mg/kg of oral midazolam in strawberry syrup preoperatively. Within 10–15 minutes, young patients will be comfortably sedated and can be taken to the operating room without difficulty. The child may be mask-induced with a mixture of oxygen and sevoflurane, an inhalational anesthetic. Every effort is made to *minimize completely* the occurrence of coughing or lid squeezing because this may increase orbital venous pressure. Once the infant or young child inhales sevoflurane, their intraocular orbital venous pressure will decrease, due to both orbital and systemic venous dilatation.

Whenever the airway is manipulated either by mask induction or placement of an oral airway, nasal airway, laryngeal mask airway, or endotracheal tube, the patient is at risk for gagging, coughing, or 'bucking.' Therefore, prior to manipulation of the patient's airway, the level of anesthesia should be sufficiently deepened during bag–mask ventilation. This will help ensure that the airway reflexes are obtunded *just* prior to instrumentation of the airway, thereby decreasing the risk of elevating intraocular pressure. Once the intravenous line is placed following a mask induction, 1–2 microgram/kg of intravenous fentanyl is administered to obtund the patient's airway reflexes, thereby preventing the patient from gagging on the endotracheal tube intraoperatively.

The infant or young child with a recent (usually within 30 days of surgery) upper URI is at increased risk for developing a highly reactive airway, manifested by bronchospasm or laryngospasm, with airway manipulation. Tracheal intubation in a patient presenting with an already increased level of airway reactivity further predisposes to the development of bronchospasm. Thus, these patients are carefully induced with general anesthesia and their level of anesthesia is deepened just prior to laryngeal manipulation.

Following glaucoma surgery, the intraocular pressure is generally lower than preoperatively. This increases the risk of suprachoroidal hemorrhage, a potentially blinding complication, if the intraocular blood pressure increases dramatically. This is most likely to occur if the patient gags or coughs during extubation.

In these instances, extubation of the patient is best performed under 'deep' general anesthesia, whereby the endotracheal tube is removed while the patient is *completely anesthetized*. Having the patient emerge from general anesthesia without the endotracheal tube in direct contact with laryngeal structures (vocal cords, aryepiglottic folds, epiglottis, laryngeal soft tissue, tongue) *minimizes* the probability of gagging, coughing, or bucking. 'Deep extubation' should only be performed in a patient who has a manageable airway, is not at risk for aspiration of gastric contents, and is able to effectively maintain spontaneous ventilation. It requires considerable experience, because performing it incorrectly will increase the risk of developing laryngospasm.

During the maintenance of general anesthesia, post-operative nausea and vomiting is mitigated by the administration of antiemetics (4 mg of IV ondansetron (Zofran) and/or 10 mg of IV metoclopramide). If a retrobulbar block was not performed intraoperatively, post-operative pain control is achieved by providing up to 2–3 microgram/kg of IV fentanyl.

POSTOPERATIVE MANAGEMENT

During the postoperative period, each patient is evaluated for his or her capacity to ventilate and oxygenate appropriately. In addition they are evaluated for pain control and level of comfort, and for the absence of nausea and/or vomiting. Patients may be discharged with an escort when their vital signs are stable, they have urinated, and are able to ambulate as well as they could preoperatively.

FURTHER READING

Cheng M, Todorov A, Tempelhoff R et al. The effect of prone positioning on intraocular pressure in anesthetized patients. Anesthesiology 2001; 95: 1351–5.

Fazio DT, Pateman JB, Christensen RE. Acute angle-closure glaucoma associated with surgical anesthesia. Arch Ophthalmol 1985; 103: 360.

Gild WM, Posner KL, Caplan RA, Cheney FW. Eye injuries associated with anesthesia: a closed claims analysis. Anesthesiology 1992; 76: 204–8.

Kelly RE, Dinner M, Turner L et al. Succinylcholine increases intraocular pressure in the human eye with the extraocular muscles detached. Anesthesiology 1993; 79: 948–52.

Kirsch RE, Samet P, Kugel V, Axelrod S. Electrocardiographic changes during ocular surgery and their prevention by retrobulbar injections. Ama Arch Ophthalmol 1957; 58: 348–56.

Lentschener C, Ghimouz A, Bonnichon P, et al. Acute post-operative glaucoma after nonocular surgery remains a diagnostic challenge. Anesth Analg 2002; 94: 1034–5.

Libonati MM, Leahy JJ, Ellison N. The use of succinylcholine in open eye surgery. Anesthesiology 1985; 62: 637–40.

Mirakhur RK, Clarke RSJ, Dundee JW, McDonald JR. Anticholinergic drugs in anesthesia. Anesthesia 1978; 33: 133–8.

Nicoll JM, Acharya PA, Ahlen K et al. Central nervous system complications after 6000 retrobulbar blocks. Anesth Analg 1987; 66: 1298–1302.

Rosenfeld SI, Litinsky SM, Snyder DA, et al. Effectiveness of monitored anesthesia care in cataract surgery. Ophthalmology 1999; 106: 1256–61.

Sator-Katzenschlager S, Deusch E, Dolezal S, et al. Sevoflurane and propofol decrease intraocular pressure equally during non-ophthalmic surgery and recovery. Br J Anesth 2002; 89: 764–6.

Siffring PA, Poulton TJ. Prevention of ophthalmic complications during general anesthesia. Anesthesiology 1987; 66: 569–70.

Sorensen EJ, Gilmore JE. Cardiac arrest during strabismus surgery. Am J Ophthalmol 1956; 41: 748.

2. Cataract surgery in patients with preexisting glaucoma

John G Ladas and Walter J Stark

INTRODUCTION

The coexistence of glaucoma and a visually significant cataract is commonly encountered in an ophthalmologic practice. The management and decision-making process for these conditions as separate entities is fairly straightforward. Cataract surgery is considered when a cataract becomes visually significant. The surgeon apprises the patient of any specific risks, and a decision to proceed with or delay surgery is made. Management of glaucoma has many options, depending on the particular type of glaucoma and the techniques available to the individual ophthalmologist. The options include medications alone, argon laser trabeculoplasty (ALT), selective laser trabeculoplasty (SLT), peripheral iridotomy, and trabeculectomy. Regardless of the method selected, glaucoma treatment will affect any future cataract surgery, and this should be factored into the decision-making process.

When a patient with glaucoma develops a visually significant cataract, the ophthalmologist must engage in important surgical decision making. The first decision to be made is whether a cataract is visually significant with respect to the underlying glaucoma. The effect of a cataract on visual function in a patient with glaucoma may include a reduction in visual field scores as well as in visual acuity. Indeed, the Advanced Glaucoma Intervention Study (AGIS) demonstrated that, on average, cataract extraction improves visual field defect scores in addition to improving visual acuity.

Once the decision to perform cataract surgery is made, the surgeon must next decide whether to proceed with cataract extraction alone, a combined cataract extraction and glaucoma procedure, or staged cataract and glaucoma procedures. Each option has its benefits and can be tailored to the individual patient. As one would expect, most studies have demonstrated that, for some patients, combined procedures result in lower final intraocular pressure (IOP) than cataract surgery alone. However, cataract surgery alone also produces long-term reductions in IOP in some patients, and this should be factored into any decision process. This chapter deals specifically with the option of cataract extraction alone in patients with preexisting glaucoma.

PREOPERATIVE EVALUATION

The ophthalmologist must consider many preoperative, perioperative, and postoperative factors for patients with cataracts and preexisting glaucoma. A thorough ophthalmologic history to determine all previous procedures is essential. In addition to ascertaining current glaucoma medications, any previous medications should also be noted. If a reduction in IOP is needed postoperatively, a particular medication response or side effect may affect the choice of medication. Finally, a thorough preoperative examination of the patient is required in order to foresee and plan for any possible intraoperative hazards. Box 2.1 provides a useful checklist for preoperative evaluation of patients with glaucoma who are considering cataract surgery.

A thorough exam can alert the surgeon to many potential intraoperative complications. Pseudoexfoliation (PXF) syndrome is hazardous, and preoperative identification of this entity is essential. Figure 2.1 shows exfoliative material on the anterior surface of a lens, with the typical 'target' appearance. This is relatively easy to diagnose, but the poor pupillary dilation sometimes associated with PXF can make the 'target' more discreet, and other signs may suggest the diagnosis.

Box 2.1 Preoperative evaluation in a patient with preexisting glaucoma

History
　Current and past medications
　Past surgeries (argon laser or selective trabeculoplasty,
　　trabeculectomy, drainage devices, peripheral iridotomy)

Exam
　Maximal dilation noted
　Anterior chamber depth
　Gonioscopy (angle architecture, peripheral synechiae)
　Pseudoexfoliation ('target', Sampaolesi line)
　Posterior synechiae
　Lens stability

Gonioscopy may reveal the Sampaolesi line, a faint pigmentation of Schwalbe's line. A diagnosis or suspicion of PXF preoperatively allows the surgeon to anticipate hazards or modify the surgical approach in specific ways, as discussed later in the chapter.

Gonioscopy is an essential part of the preoperative work-up of these patients. Specifically, narrow angles and shallow anterior chamber are noted, as well as peripheral synechiae, such as in a patient with previous neovascular glaucoma. Eyes with an extremely shallow anterior chamber may have a phacomorphic component to the elevated IOP. Peripheral iridotomies and medications can control the pressure in the preoperative period, but intraoperatively these eyes can present a difficult challenge, with an increased risk of corneal decompensation or suprachoroidal hemorrhage. A pars plana vitrectomy to deepen the anterior chamber may be necessary if adequate chamber depth to perform phacoemulsification cannot be obtained to allow the surgeon to proceed safely with cataract surgery.

Some less common circumstances may also be encountered during cataract surgery in patients with glaucoma. Figure 2.2 shows a mature white cataract. In addition to poor visibility of the anterior capsule in such a case, the potential for weak zonules and the need for prolonged phacoemulsification time should be anticipated.

Instability of the zonules may be difficult to ascertain preoperatively, but a few methods can detect its presence. A gentle tap on the slit lamp while observing the lens can reveal increased lens mobility. Although rare, some patients with PXF may have observable zonular loss and vitreous in the anterior chamber. A vitrectomy, from an anterior or posterior approach, can be planned, as well as potential methods to suture an intraocular lens can be formulated by making this diagnosis preoperatively.

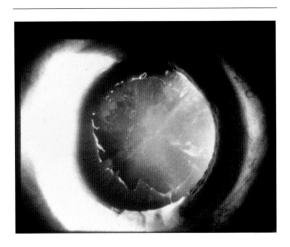

Figure 2.1 Pseudoexfoliation of a lens capsule.

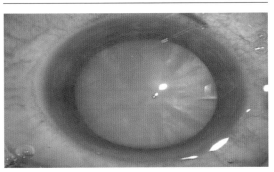

Figure 2.2 A mature white cataract.

ROLE OF PRIOR ARGON LASER TRABECULOPLASTY

A significant number of patients with glaucoma and visually significant cataracts have undergone prior ALT. There is little information on the effect of subsequent cataract surgery on IOP in these patients. One study suggested a possible increase in IOP immediately after cataract surgery in eyes with prior ALT. This study demonstrated that an IOP increase of more than 10 mmHg on the day after surgery occurred in significantly more patients previously treated with ALT than in patients who were medically treated for glaucoma. The potential mechanism behind this finding is unclear, but these patients may need closer follow-up and short-term management of pressure control after cataract surgery.

Other studies have shown that the IOP reduction achieved after ALT is not diminished after subsequent cataract surgery. In our experience, prior ALT does not alter the routine postoperative course of cataract surgery.

SHORT- AND LONG-TERM EFFECTS OF CATARACT SURGERY ON INTRAOCULAR PRESSURE

Most studies have shown that IOP decreases after phacoemulsification cataract surgery. The IOP in the immediate postoperative period in glaucomatous and nonglaucomatous eyes may be lower than anticipated, but is within normal range in most patients 1 day after surgery. Shingleton and colleagues (2001) showed that a significant number of eyes exhibited hypotony (IOP < 5 mmHg) 30 minutes after cataract surgery, but these returned to normal levels by 1 day postoperatively. There is also some evidence that extracapsular cataract extraction may temporarily elevate the IOP in the short term. In addition, previous ALT may affect IOP, as described above.

The long-term reduction in IOP following cataract surgery is of the order of 2–4 mmHg, and occurs in the majority of patients. Indeed, studies have demonstrated that clear corneal phacoemulsification resulted in lower IOP 1 year after surgery in patients with no glaucoma, patients with glaucoma, or patients suspected of having glaucoma. Also, some evidence suggests that the long-term reduction may be greater in patients with a history of angle closure glaucoma than in those with open angle glaucoma. Thus, regardless of the type of glaucoma, there seems to be a long-term lowering of IOP following clear corneal phacoemulsification.

This reduction of IOP appears to be independent of the presence of pseudoexfoliation. A study by Pohjalainen and colleagues (2001) showed that while pressure spikes may be more common in patients with PXF on the first postoperative day, long-term pressure reduction occurred in all patients undergoing cataract surgery, from 1 week to more than 1 year after surgery. The authors have observed an IOP reduction of more than 20% in eyes with and without PXF more than 1 year after cataract surgery. This is in agreement with other studies that have reported a greater long-term IOP reduction in patients with PXF.

This effect on IOP should be anticipated in patients with glaucoma and cataracts. In one study, 34% of patients with preexisting glaucoma no longer required glaucoma medications 1 year after phacoemulsification alone. While the magnitude of the IOP reduction may be relatively small, the surgeon should factor this into the glaucoma management of a particular patient. For instance, for a patient with glaucoma and a coexisting cataract who is being considered for implementation of IOP medications, the decision may be to do the cataract surgery first and establish a new IOP baseline. The small reduction in IOP after cataract surgery may be sufficient to warrant observation of the patient, without introduction of a new medication. Also, in a patient whose IOP has been kept stable by medication for many years but who has now developed a cataract there might be, after surgery, a reduction in IOP that will maintain the pressure below target level in the absence of additional or any glaucoma medications.

There is some evidence to suggest that the size of the capsulorhexis may affect early postoperative IOP, with a smaller capsulorhexis leading to a lower IOP. However, no difference in the long-term effect is apparent.

The long-term management of IOP in patients with glaucoma after cataract surgery is essentially the same as prior to surgery. The ophthalmologist has the option of prescribing any of the available medications or performing procedures such as ALT or trabeculectomy. In the short term, fluctuations in IOP can be managed with aqueous suppressants.

SURGICAL APPROACH

There are many techniques for cataract extraction in patients with glaucoma, but we routinely use a temporal or nasal clear corneal approach to avoid damage to the conjunctiva, which may be needed for future procedures. A standard set of surgical instruments is used for routine cataracts, and some instruments and devices are available for use in special circumstances (Box 2.2).

Iris retractors can be particularly helpful to enlarge a miotic pupil which may be found in patients with pseudoexfoliation syndrome. Four retractors are sufficient in most cases, but there are times when five may prove useful. Other devices to enlarge a miotic pupil are available, but based on our experience and the ease of use, we prefer the iris retractor.

STEP-BY-STEP GUIDE

Of the many ways to perform cataract surgery on patients with glaucoma, we describe here our preferred technique.

The eye is dilated with three sets of cyclopentolate 1%, tropicamide 1%, and phenylephrine hydrochloride (Neosynephrine) 2.5%. After adequate dilation of at least 5 mm (Figure 2.3), topical xylocaine jelly 2% is applied. Generally, with a dilation of less than 5 mm, we consider enlarging the pupil using methods described below.

> **Box 2.2 Surgical instruments for cataract extraction**
>
> **Standard instruments**
>   Keratome or diamond knife
>   Supersharp blade
>   Viscoelastic agent
>   Capsular forceps
>   Second instrument (nucleus chopper, lens spatula)
>   Phacoemulsification unit
>   Lens inserter or lens forceps
>
> **Special instruments**
>   Iris retractors
>   Long-angled Vannas scissors
>   Indocyanine dye
>   10-0 Prolene suture on a CTC needle (Ethicon)

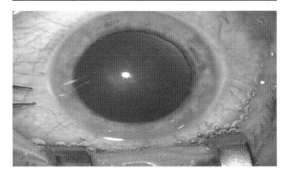

Figure 2.3 Good dilation and red reflex.

A clear corneal incision is made at the steep axis of corneal astigmatism, unless the location is limited by a preexisting trabeculectomy. We make a linear epithelial incision with the tip of the diamond knife at the limbus (Figure 2.4) and penetrate the anterior chamber with the diamond blade, using a biplanar incision of at least 2.5 mm (Figure 2.5). The anterior chamber is then filled with a cohesive viscoelastic agent to provide adequate tension on the anterior capsule. This is particularly important if the patient has a 'floppy' capsule, as observed in some patients with PXF.

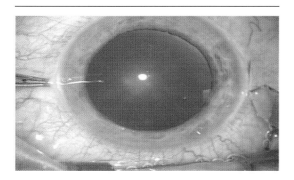

Figure 2.4 The epithelial incision.

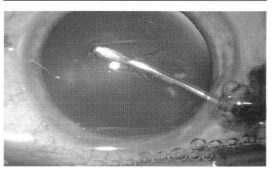

Figure 2.6 The creation of an anterior capsular tear.

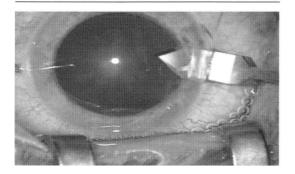

Figure 2.5 Entry into the anterior chamber.

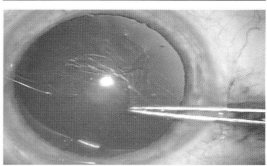

Figure 2.7 Creating the capsulorhexis.

A cystotome is used to create an anterior capsular tear (Figure 2.6). Careful observation of the dynamics of the anterior capsule as the cystotome creates the tear can help the surgeon detect potential zonular instability. Capsular forceps are then used to create a continuous curvilinear capsulorhexis (Figure 2.7). We prefer a large capsulorhexis, of the order of 6–6.5 mm. This allows for thorough hydrodissection and nucleus mobility during the procedure. Hydrodissection and hydrodelineation are then performed using a 25-gauge cannula, until the lens prolapses out of the bag or good nuclear mobility is noted (Figure 2.8).

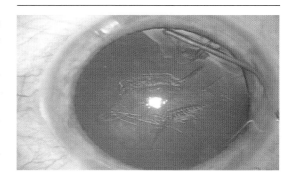

Figure 2.8 Hydrodissection.

This can be particularly helpful in patients with PXF and zonular instability; the surgeon can thus perform the majority of the phacoemulsification in the iris plane rather than in the capsular bag which reduces the stress on the zonules.

If the patient has coexisting endothelial dystrophy, a dispersive viscoelastic agent that remains throughout the phacoemulsification, such as Viscoat (Alcon Laboratories), can be used in a soft shell technique. Approximately 0.1 ml of the viscoelastic is layered below the endothelium prior to phacoemulsification.

A central groove is created using the phacoemulsification unit (Figure 2.9). Orientation of the second instrument and the phacoemulsification handpiece 180° apart gives the surgeon excellent control of the eye, which is particularly helpful when the patient has been given topical anesthesia. Once the central groove is of adequate depth, the nucleus is split (Figure 2.10) and the individual halves removed (Figure 2.11).

After irrigation and aspiration of the remaining cortical material, the capsular bag is reinflated with the viscoelastic agent (Figure 2.12a). If needed, the clear corneal incision is enlarged and the intraocular lens is placed in the capsular bag (Figure 2.12 b,c). We generally use an acrylic lens, implanted with an inserter or use a lens forceps with the lens folded in a 'moustache' fold. The lens is then posi-

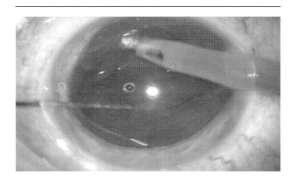

Figure 2.10 Splitting the nucleus.

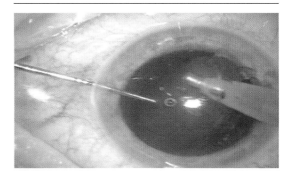

Figure 2.11 Removal of the individual halves.

tioned centrally (Figure 2.13). The viscoelastic agent is removed with the irrigation and aspiration handpiece (Figure 2.14). Complete removal of the viscoelastic agent at the end of the procedure is important to reduce the potential for postoperative elevation in IOP, which could be damaging for patients with advanced glaucoma.

MANAGEMENT OF INTRAOPERATIVE HAZARDS: SPECIAL TECHNIQUES

In cataract surgery on patients with preexisting glaucoma, certain situations may arise that warrant mention here. First, a good clear corneal wound of adequate length is important, particularly in eyes

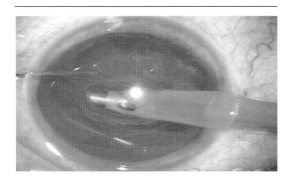

Figure 2.9 The central groove.

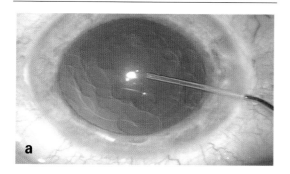

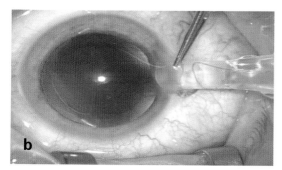

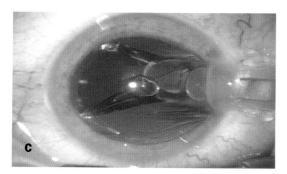

Figures 2.12 (a–c) Insertion of the lens.

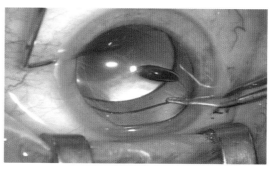

Figure 2.13 Positioning the lens.

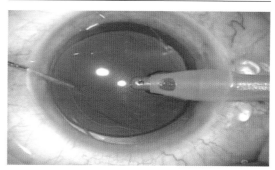

Figure 2.14 Removal of the viscoelastic agent.

with narrow angles or with a 'floppy iris' that may enter an inadequate wound during the procedure. If the iris does prolapse through the wound during phacoemulsification, delicate repositioning of the iris may be performed with or without the use of a viscoelastic agent. Should this fail, the surgeon could consider a peripheral iridectomy to help reposition the iris.

Patients with preexisting pseudoexfoliative glaucoma have a higher risk than other cataract patients of zonular weakness and vitreous loss during the procedure. If vitreous loss is encountered intraoperatively, a thorough anterior vitrectomy is essential for two reasons: vitreous in the anterior chamber may elevate the pressure in the short term and may complicate future filtering procedures. If vitreous loss does occur during the procedure, we place a sulcus intraocular lens, provided there is enough anterior capsular support. It is important to use a lens with a large optic, at least 6–6.5 mm, to decrease the risk of further prolapse into the anterior chamber. Occasionally, in patients with extremely weak zonules, an actual dehiscence may occur during the procedure. We prefer to place the intraocular lens within the capsular bag if there is enough capsular support to maintain it in position – usually less than about 2 clock hours of complete zonular dehiscence. In the absence of sufficient capsular support, the lens can be placed in the sulcus or iris fixated, using techniques described below.

Other situations requiring special intraoperative techniques include eyes with unique anatomic characteristics, a previous history of trauma, underlying systemic disease, or previous ophthalmic surgery.

'White' or mature cataracts can present particular difficulties for the cataract surgeon (Figure 2.15). If the cataract is mature, increased phacoemulsification power is typically needed during the procedure, which requires special attention to preservation of the endothelium by using a dispersive viscoelastic agent in a soft shell technique. A white cataract can also occur with preexisting trauma, and in such cases attention to zonular stability is required during surgery. These two situations may be anticipated with a thorough preoperative history.

Regardless of the technique used, the most challenging part of the procedure is typically the capsulorhexis. In the absence of a good red reflex, we use an intracameral dye to stain the anterior capsule prior to the capsulorhexis. Many dyes have been described in the literature, but our preference is indocyanine green (ICG). The ICG is diluted as described by Horiguchi et al. (1998) and in Chapter 6 of this book. After creation of a clear corneal incision, the aqueous is replaced with an air bubble (Figures 2.16, 2.17). A few drops of dilute ICG are placed on the anterior capsule and lightly dispersed with a cannula (Figure 2.18). The air bubble in the anterior chamber is then replaced with a cohesive viscoelastic agent. Next, a capsulorhexis is performed, as usual, with good visualization of the anterior capsule against the white cataract (Figure 2.19), followed by hydrodissection and hydrodelineation. During phacoemulsification, the surgeon should pay particular attention to the density of the lens, particularly in eyes with mature cataracts, which may lack an epinucleus that protects the pos-

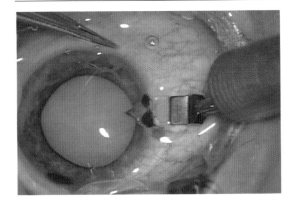

Figure 2.16 Clear corneal incision.

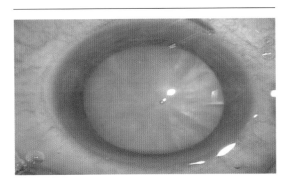

Figure 2.15 Mature white cataract.

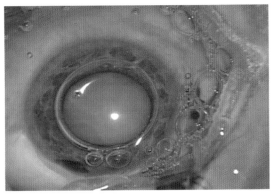

Figure 2.17 Replacement of aqueous with an air bubble.

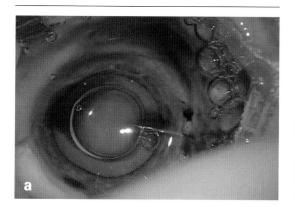

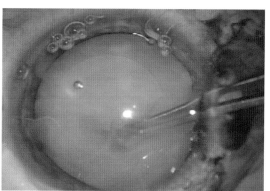

Figure 2.19 Capsulorhexis under good visualization.

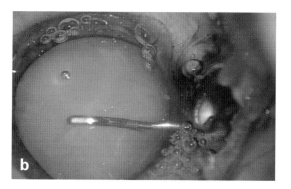

Figure 2.18 (a,b) Indocyanine dye instilled onto the anterior capsule and is replaced with viscoelastic.

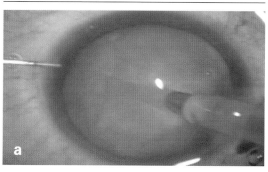

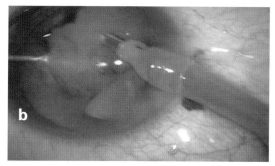

Figure 2.20 (a, b) Phacoemulsification of white cataract.

terior capsule during phacoemulsification and chop techniques (Figure 2.20 a,b).

Narrow anatomic angles present particular challenges during cataract surgery. The first consideration in these patients is whether they have preexisting iridotomies. Sometimes it can be beneficial to make the clear corneal incision in the same clock hour as the iridotomy; this may prevent prolapse of the iris through the incision during surgery. Attention must also be paid to constructing a wound of the proper transcorneal length, again to prevent prolapse of the iris during surgery.

Another special situation that requires both preoperative planning and specific intraoperative techniques is phacodonesis. This condition can result from ocular trauma or PXF. If phacodonesis is diagnosed preoperatively, the surgeon can anticipate complications and prepare to use special instru-

ments. The first intraoperative challenge in these patients is the capsulorhexis. Irregular zonular tension may result in irregular tearing of the capsulorhexis. We pay close attention to ensure that the flap is folded on itself as the capsulorhexis is performed. If this is not done, radialization or extension can occur as the surgeon encounters different capsular forces. We also closely observe the overall stability of the lens. If the lens seems very unstable, capsular retention hooks may be placed – two to four hooks in the area of zonular instability. This technique works only with an intact capsulorhexis. Once the capsular hooks are in place, hydrodissection is performed and phacoemulsification can proceed.

Once the cataract is removed, we evaluate the capsular bag to determine whether it can support an intraocular lens. We prefer to place the lens in the capsular bag if there is enough capsular support. A bag with zonular instability in an inferior location may tolerate an intracapsular lens better than one with instability in a superior position. If there is not enough capsular stability within the bag, however, the lens can be placed in the sulcus, provided there is enough stability. We use a large optic lens of at least 6.5 mm. When capsular support is inadequate, various methods can be used to suture-fixate the intraocular lens. Compared with transcleral fixation we feel suture fixation to the mid-peripheral iris using a foldable lens is less traumatic and less likely to result in a 'tilted' lens postoperatively.

The technique for implanting a foldable intraocular lens in the absence of capsular support has been described elsewhere. The first step is to fill the anterior chamber with a cohesive viscoelastic agent (Figure 2.21). Next, the lens is folded in a 'moustache' configuration (Figure 2.22a,b) and inserted into the eye through the clear corneal incision. The haptics are then oriented posteriorly, and a second instrument such as a cyclodialysis spatula is inserted 180° from the clear corneal wound (Figure 2.23) and delicately placed below the lens optic. The lens is allowed to unfold as the second instrument supports it (Figure 2.24). Pupillary capture of the optic is achieved by instilling acetylcholine chloride (Miochol).

The lens is now in position to suture-fixate it to the iris. A 10-0 Prolene suture on a CTC needle is inserted at the limbus (Figure 2.25a), through the iris and below the haptic (Figure 2.25b), and back

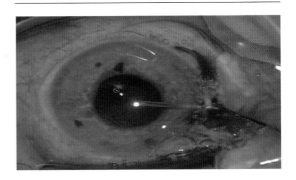

Figure 2.21 Forming the anterior chamber.

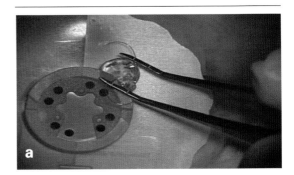

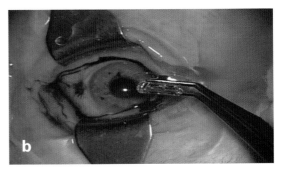

Figure 2.22 (a, b) Preparing the foldable lens in a 'moustache' configuration.

through the limbus (Figure 2.25c). The same maneuver is performed with the opposite haptic (Figure 2.26). Stab incisions are made at the limbus equidistant from the individual passes of the 10-0 Prolene. The sutures are then retrieved through the stab incisions and temporarily tied using a modified McCannel technique (Figure 2.27). The lens is then

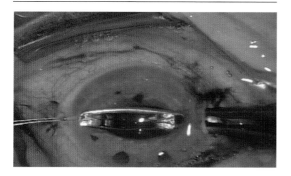

Figure 2.23 Placement of the spatula.

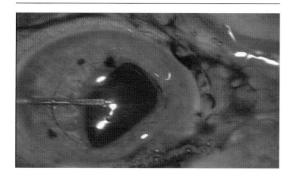

Figure 2.24 Supporting the lens as it unfolds.

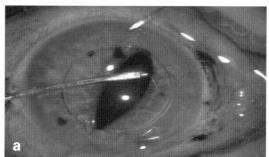

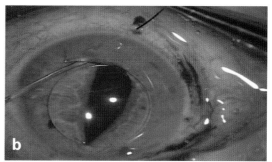

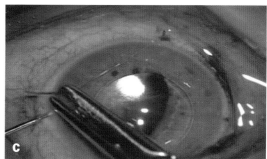

Figure 2.25 (a–c) Placement of Prolene supporting sutures.

gently placed into the posterior chamber (Figure 2.28) and, after ensuring that the pupil is round and central, the sutures are permanently tied (Figure 2.29). An air bubble is then placed in the anterior chamber, and the chamber swept with a spatula to ensure no vitreous remains (Figure 2.30). The air bubble is removed and the anterior chamber is filled with a balanced salt solution (Figure 2.31).

Another special situation arises when the pupil needs to be enlarged prior to cataract surgery. Although pupil stretching techniques and sphincterectomies have been described, our preferred technique, as shown in a case of PXF and persistent miosis (Figure 2.32a), is the use of iris retractors.

After creation of the clear corneal incision and placement of a viscoelastic agent in the anterior chamber, four or five limbal stab incisions are made (Figures 2.32b, c). If four retractors are to be used,

the stab incisions are made 90° apart and away from the corneal incision. We find it beneficial to direct the stab incisions posteriorly (toward the iris) rather than toward the center of the pupil. This allows the iris retractors to stretch the iris and maintain it in a posterior position, as opposed to being tented anteriorly, during the procedure. Each retractor is inserted (Figure 2.33a) and the iris margin is engaged with the hook (Figure 2.33b). This is done for each of the four retractors (Figure

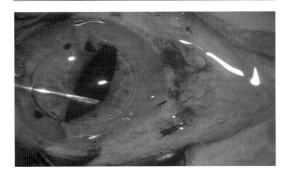

Figure 2.26 Placement of the Prolene supporting sutures.

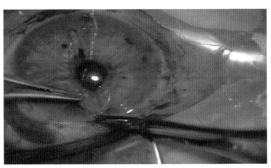

Figure 2.29 Permanent fixation of sutures.

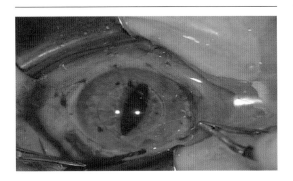

Figure 2.27 Tying the sutures.

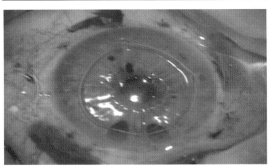

Figure 2.30 Using an air bubble to check for vitreous.

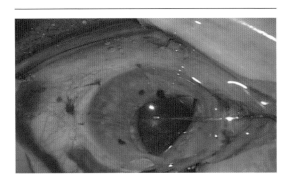

Figure 2.28 Placement of the lens in the posterior chamber.

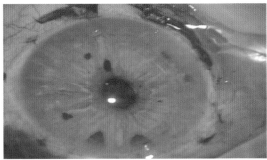

Figure 2.31 Replacing the air bubble with balanced salt solution.

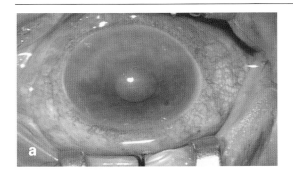

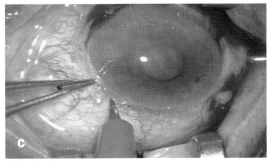

Figure 2.32 (a) Miotic pupil. (b, c) Stab incision for placement of retractors.

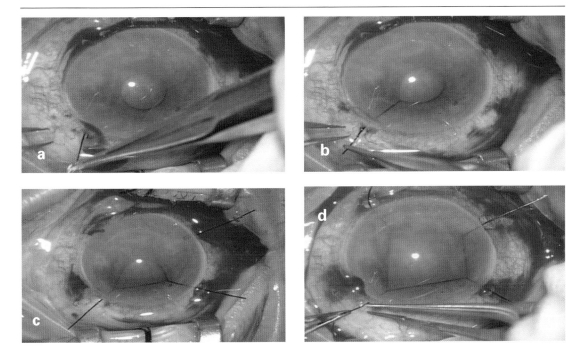

Figures 2.33 (a–d) Placement of retractors.

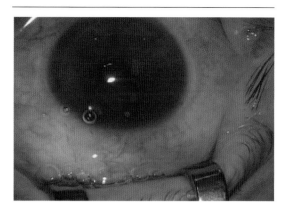

Figure 2.34 Cataract miosis in a patient with a preexisting bleb with a miotic pupil.

2.33c), and the silicon sleeve of the retractor is moved to lock the retractor and iris into an enlarged position (Figure 2.33). After the cataract is extracted and the intraocular lens placed, the iris retractors are removed by first moving the silicon sleeve and then disengaging the hook from the iris. Each retractor can then be removed from the eye. This is done prior to removing the viscoelastic.

Other special situations involve eyes that have undergone previous surgery. In patients with a preexisting drainage device, such as an Ahmed or Baerveldt valve, a clear corneal incision is placed away from the drainage device. Given their location, drainage devices are typically not obstructive

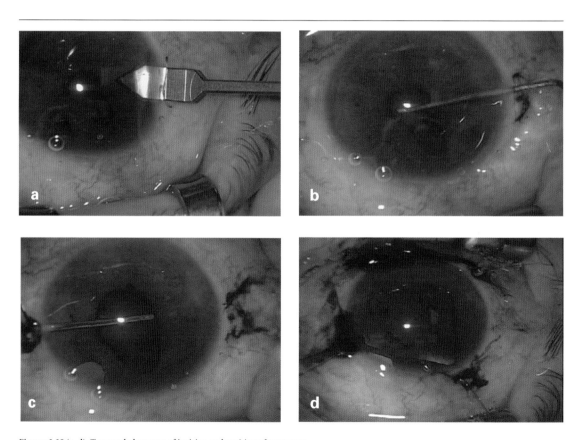

Figures 2.35 (a–d) Temporal placement of incision and position of retractors.

to cataract surgery. In patients with prior trabeculectomies, we perform our cataract extraction
with a clear corneal technique, using a location
away from an existing trabeculectomy site, as in the
case of a patient with a functioning bleb and posterior synechiae (Figure 2.34). We avoid damaging
the conjunctiva during the procedure by handling
the conjunctiva as far from the bleb as possible
Making the incisions temporally and nasally is particularly beneficial in these patients (Figure 2.35a).
After instillation of a viscoelastic agent, the posterior synechiae can be gently dissected from both
incisions (Figures 2.35b,c). Iris retractors can than
be placed, as previously described, to allow for
adequate dilation (Figure 2.35d).

CONCLUSIONS

Performing cataract surgery in patients with preexisting glaucoma is a common occurrence in ophthalmology. A thorough preoperative evaluation is
important in determining the best method for surgery and in preparing the surgeon for any possible
intraoperative hazards. A few specialized techniques can ensure good outcomes when adverse
intraoperative events occur in these sometimes
complicated eyes.

FURTHER READING

AGIS Investigators. The advanced glaucoma intervention study. 6: Effect of cataract on visual field and visual acuity. Arch Ophthalmol 2000; 118: 1639–52.

Brown SV, Thomas JV, Budenz DL, Bellows AR, Simmons RJ. Effect of cataract surgery on intraocular pressure reduction with laser trabeculoplasty. Am J Ophthalmol 1985; 100: 373–6.

Calissendorff BM, Hamberg-Nystrom H. Pressure control in glaucoma patients after cataract surgery with intraocular lens. Eur J Ophthalmol 1992; 2: 163–8.

Cekic O, Batman C. Effect of capsulorhexis size on postoperative intraocular pressure. J Cataract Refract Surg 1999; 25: 416–19.

Chang DF. Pars plana vitrectomy tap for phacoemulsification in the crowded eye. J Cataract Refract Surg 2001; 27: 1911–14.

Cinotti DJ, Fiore PM, Maltzman BA, Constad WH, Cinotti AA. Control of intraocular pressure in glaucomatous eyes after extracapsular cataract extraction with intraocular lens implantation. J Cataract Refract Surg 1988; 14: 650–3.

Dimitrov PN, Mukesh BN, Taylor HR, McCarty CA. Intraocular pressure before and after cataract surgery in participants of the Melbourne Visual Impairment Project. Clin Exp Ophthalmol 2001; 29: 128–32.

Freissler K, Kuchle M, Naumann GO. Spontaneous dislocation of the lens in pseudoexfoliation syndrome. Ophthalmology 1995; 113: 1095–6.

Friedman DS, Jampel HD Lubomski LH, et al. Surgical strategies for coexisting glaucoma and cataract: an evidence-based update. Ophthalmology 2002; 109: 1902–15.

Horiguchi M, Miyake K, Ohta I, Ito Y. Staining of the lens capsule for circular continuous capsulorhexis in eyes with white cataract. Arch Ophthalmol 1998; 116: 535–7.

Kuchle M, Viestenz A, Martus P et al. Anterior chamber depth and complications during cataract surgery in eyes with pseudoexfoliation syndrome. Am J Ophthalmol 2000; 129: 281–5.

McGuigan LJ, Gottsch J, Stark WJ et al. Extracapsular cataract extraction and posterior chamber lens implantation in eyes with preexisting glaucoma. Arch Ophthalmol 1986; 104: 1301–8.

Merkur A, Damji KF, Mintsioulis G, Hodge WG. Intraocular pressure decrease after phacoemulsification in patients with pseudoexfoliation syndrome. J Cataract Refract Surg 2001; 27: 528–32.

Perasalo R. Phacoemulsification of cataract in eyes with glaucoma. Acta Ophthalmol Scand 1997; 75: 299–300.

Pohjalainen T, Vesti E, Uusitalo RJ, Laatikainen L. Phacoemulsification and intraocular lens implantation in eyes with open-angle glaucoma. Acta Ophthalmol Scand 2001; 79: 313–16.

Pohjalainen T, Vesti E, Uusitalo RJ, Laatikainen L. Intraocular pressure after phacoemulsification and intraocular lens implantation in nonglaucomatous eyes with and without exfoliation. J Cataract Refract Surg 2001; 27: 426–31.

Shingleton BJ, Gamell LS, O'Donoghue MW, Baylus SL, King R. Long-term changes in intraocular pressure changes after clear corneal phacoemulsification: normal patients versus glaucoma suspect and glaucoma patients. J Cataract Refract Surg 1999; 25: 885–90.

Shingleton BJ, Wadhwani RA, O'Donoghue MW, Baylus S, Hoey H. Evaluation of intraocular pressure in the immediate period after phacoemulsification. J Cataract Refract Surg 2001; 27: 524–7.

Snyder ME. Pseudoexfoliation and cataract surgery. Rev Ophthalmol 2001; Sep: 31–8.

Stutzman R, Stark WJ. Surgical technique for suture fixation of an acrylic intraocular lens in the absence of capsule support. J Cataract Ref Surg 2003; 29: 1658–62.

3. Trabeculectomy

Keith Barton

INTRODUCTION

In patients with both uncontrolled glaucoma and visually significant cataract, trabeculectomy alone may in certain circumstances be more appropriate than either a combined phacoemulsification and filtration surgery or phacoemulsification alone.

SITUATIONS IN WHICH TRABECULECTOMY ALONE MAY BE APPROPRIATE

Clearly, a prerequisite for glaucoma surgery prior to cataract surgery is loss of intraocular pressure (IOP) control on the maximum tolerated level of medication. The indications for glaucoma filtration surgery alone fall loosely into three categories:

1. When a large IOP drop or low postoperative IOP level are desirable.
2. When the prognosis for IOP control with combined surgery is poor because of excessive conjunctival scarring or the presence of a secondary glaucoma.
3. When phacoemulsification may be complicated, reducing the prospect of trabeculectomy success.

WHERE A LARGE IOP DROP OR LOW POSTOPERATIVE IOP ARE DESIRABLE

Patients who require a large IOP drop because either the preoperative IOP is very high or a low postoperative IOP is required (advanced glaucomatous optic neuropathy or normal pressure glaucoma) may be considered in this category.

The author's preference for filtration surgery performed in isolation is based on the greater degree of IOP reduction that can be achieved by this approach, when compared with phacotrabeculectomy. When surgery is required for uncontrolled glaucoma in the presence of a visually significant cataract, the primary aim is IOP control. Phacotrabeculectomy compared head to head with trabeculectomy has been reported to have 40–60% (4–6 mmHg) less IOP-lowering effect than trabeculectomy alone. Although often this may be sufficient, a low target IOP is more likely to be achieved with trabeculectomy alone.

SECONDARY GLAUCOMAS AND CONJUNCTIVAL SCARRING

In certain secondary glaucomas, for instance uveitic glaucoma, trabeculectomy with antiproliferative agents is even less likely to control the IOP when combined with cataract surgery. Anterior segment and conjunctival inflammation are greater after a combined procedure than after trabeculectomy alone, lowering the chances of filtration success. A concomitant reduction in aqueous production in patients with chronic inflammation further compromises filtration success by limiting bleb formation in the early postoperative period. Finally, postoperative overdrainage of a filtration bleb after phacotrabeculectomy in the uveitic may result, not only in IOL-pupil capture but also excessive fibrin deposition due to the combined effects of hypotony and a compromised blood-aqueous barrier. Trabeculectomy success is therefore optimized in uveitic patients by avoiding simultaneous cataract surgery.

In other types of secondary glaucoma such as aphakic and post-keratoplasty glaucoma, iridocorneal endothelial (ICE) syndrome, neovascular glaucoma, epithelial downgrowth and silicone oil-related secondary open angle glaucoma, the prognosis for trabeculectomy, even with mitomycin, is poor and other forms of surgical management such as drainage implant surgery or cyclophotocoagulation should be considered.

WHEN CATARACT SURGERY MIGHT BE COMPLICATED

If cataract surgery is likely to be complicated by vitreous loss, e.g. poor zonular support in pseudo-exfoliation syndrome, or where an additional manipulation such as IOL suturing might be required, the extra manipulation may compromise trabeculectomy success. Cataract surgery involving extra manipulation creates the potential for excessive postoperative inflammation or even sclerostomy blockage with vitreous. If this can be anticipated, then trabeculectomy alone is more likely to succeed in controlling IOP.

POTENTIAL NEGATIVE ASPECTS OF TRABECULECTOMY ALONE

While a trabeculectomy alone may achieve better IOP control than a phacotrabeculectomy, some of this advantage is negated by a subsequent phacoemulsification. When a visually significant cataract exists at the time of a trabeculectomy, later cataract surgery is almost inevitable. Approximately 30% of primary open angle glaucoma trabeculectomies will lose IOP control after a subsequent cataract surgery. When a cataract exists preoperatively but is not yet visually significant, a trabeculectomy in isolation is also likely to accelerate cataract formation and increase the likelihood of future cataract surgery.

SURGICAL APPROACH

LIST OF SURGICAL INSTRUMENTS

See Table 3.1 for a list of instruments required for trabeculectomy.

SURGICAL PRINCIPLES – TRABECULECTOMY SITE

The exact site for the trabeculectomy requires consideration. Inappropriate choice of a site can result in an interpalpebral or exposure zone bleb and postoperative complications such as dysesthesia and infection. The best place for a trabeculectomy is at the 12 o'clock position. This minimizes the risk of aqueous tracking nasally or temporally into the interpalpebral subconjunctival space.

In certain situations the 12 o'clock position may be unavailable. Large anterior ciliary vessels may perforate the sclera too close to the limbus for it to be possible to fashion a flap, or there may be superior conjunctival scarring from a previous trabeculectomy. As repeat trabeculectomies generally require the use of mitomycin C (MMC), the position of the trabeculectomy is an important consideration. The author's preferred practice is to operate as close to 12 o'clock as is practical, and to endeavor to apply MMC at 12 o'clock in a wide area posterior to the previous site. If a trabeculectomy is to be performed off the 12 o'clock axis, then temporal is preferable to nasal in order to prevent later dysesthesia. Placement of MMC in the superior fornix will encourage aqueous to track posteriorly rather than circumferentially. The surgeon will then have minimized the risk of producing an exposure zone bleb (a bleb in the interpalpebral area).

If a repeat trabeculectomy is deemed necessary, but no suitable adjacent site is available, then drainage device implantation or cyclophotocoagulation may be more appropriate.

SURGICAL PRINCIPLES – FORNIX VERSUS LIMBUS-BASED CONJUNCTIVAL FLAPS

The aim of filtration surgery is to control the IOP by means of a guarded sclerostomy that restricts aqueous flow into the subconjunctival space. Aqueous is then absorbed from the subconjunctival space either by absorption into the lymphatic and vascular system or by transconjunctival 'sweating'. In a successful trabeculectomy, the point of maximal resistance to outflow is the scleral flap,

Table 3.1 Surgical instruments for trabeculectomy

Instrument	Comment
Conjunctival dissection	
Westcott scissors	Duckworth and Kent, St Louis, MO, USA
Microsurgical forceps	Both grooved and plain; Duckworth and Kent, St Louis, MO, USA
Diathermy	Eraser – 20-gauge disposable bipolar pencil; Kirwan Surgical Products, Marshfield, MA, USA
	or
	Forceps; Storz Ophthalmics, St Louis, MO, USA
Mitomycin C (MMC) application	Use nonfragmenting sponges (e.g. PVA sponges such as corneal light shields); Merocel Corneal Light Shields, Solan, Xomed Surgical Products, Jacksonville, FL, USA
MMC	Kyowa Hakko Kogyo Co Ltd, Tokyo, Japan
	or
	Mutamycin, Bristol-Myers-Squibb, New York, New York, USA
5-Fluorouracil	50 mg/ml; Faulding Pharmaceuticals PLC, Mulgrave, Victoria, Australia
Knives	
Clearing episclera and Tenon's capsule	
Tooks knife	Duckworth and Kent, St. Louis, MO, USA
Scleral flap	30-degree blade; Microfeather Ophthalmic Scalpel, Medical Division, Feather Safety Razor Company, Japan
	Crescent knife and 3.2-mm slit knife, 20-degree V-lance
	or
	Beaver 69 and 75 blades; Alcon Laboratories Inc., Fort Worth, TX, USA
Paracentesis	30-degree blade; Microfeather Ophthalmic Scalpel, see above
	or
	Grieshaber 20-gauge blade; Grieshaber, Schaffhausen, Switzerland
	MVR blade, 20-gauge; Alcon, Fort Worth, Texas
	or
	Beaver 75 blade.
	In the author's practice a feather blade is used (see above)
Descemet's punch	Luntz-Dodick; Katena Products Inc., Denville, NJ, USA
	Kelly; Duckworth and Kent, St Louis, MO, USA
Peripheral iridectomy	De Weckers or Vannas scissors; Duckworth and Kent, St Louis, MO, USA
Rycroft cannula	30-gauge anterior chamber ophthalmic cannula; Steriseal, Maersk Medical Inc., McAllen, Texas, USA
Needle holders and sutures	Microsurgical needle holders; Duckworth and Kent, St Louis, MO, USA
	Corneal traction suture – 7-0 silk; Ethicon, Johnson and Johnson International, Brussels, Belgium
	10-0 nylon for scleral flap and conjunctiva; Alcon Laboratories Inc., Fort Worth, TX, USA
	or
	10-0 Vicryl for conjunctiva; Ethicon, Johnson and Johnson International, Brussels, Belgium (spatulated needle)
Fluids	
Irrigating fluid for removal of MMC afterwards	Aqsia intraocular irrigating soution (Chauvin, Labege, France)
Viscoelastic	Healon; Pfizer, New York, NY, USA
	or
	Provisc; Alcon Laboratories Inc., Fort Worth, TX, USA
Subconjunctival antibiotics	Cefuroxime (Zinacef; Glaxo Operations UK, Greenford, Middlesex, UK)
	Betamethasone sodium phosphate (Betnesol; Celltech Pharmaceuticals Limited, Slough, UK)

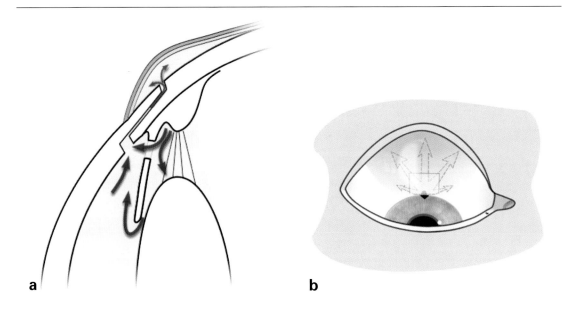

Figure 3.1 (a,b) The ideal drainage bleb is diffuse and situated posterior to the scleral flap.

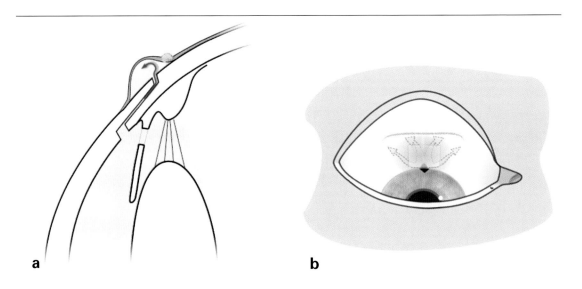

Figure 3.2 (a,b) The posterior conjunctival entry site for the limbus-based flap often induces extensive subconjunctival scarring forming a posterior barrier to aqueous diffusion and restricting bleb formation to the perilimbal conjunctiva.

and the conjunctival drainage bleb is a low-pressure aqueous reservoir which should have sufficient capacity to permit an adequate rate of aqueous absorption or transconjunctival flow. To achieve this, the surgeon must be able to close the scleral wound tightly to restrict aqueous flow in the early postoperative period to prevent early hypotony, while simultaneously preserving the ability to regulate scleral resistance by loosening the flap later.

For the scleral flap to function as the main pressure regulator, the subconjunctival space must have a capacity for aqueous absorption which can match the rate of delivery of aqueous through the sclerostomy. The limiting factor in achieving this is often subconjunctival scarring. Trabeculectomy surgery should aim to induce as little scarring as possible in the postoperative subconjunctival space and the ideal drainage bleb should be low in elevation and diffuse with low potential for postoperative dysesthesia and infection (Figure 3.1).

The method of conjunctival entry has an important effect on the postoperative behaviour of the bleb. The limbus-based conjunctival flap has been popular when performing antiproliferative trabeculectomies because of the ease of achieving watertight closure, with lower risk of early postoperative bleb leakage. Despite this obvious advantage, the present author prefers the fornix-based conjunctival flap because the resultant bleb morphology is better and the likelihood of long-term

complications is probably lower. The early bleb leakage, which has limited the widespread popularity of the fornix-based conjunctival flap, is a risk factor for late bleb failure, but can usually be avoided by careful attention to conjunctival closure. On the other hand the conjunctival incision of the limbus-based flap typically results in a scar that demarcates the bleb posteriorly, impeding posterior drainage of aqueous through the subconjunctival space and limiting the bleb to the perilimbal area (Figure 3.2). Limbus-based flaps therefore create blebs that are more anteriorly placed and more focal than those that can be achieved by the fornix-based flap (Figure 3.3). Interestingly, neither type of flap appears to confer better IOP control.

SURGICAL PRINCIPLES – USE OF ANTIMETABOLITES

A trabeculectomy may fail to reduce the IOP to an acceptable level because of resistance to aqueous outflow at one or more sites in the outflow pathway (Figure 3.4). Blockage of the internal osteum is relatively uncommon and usually preventable with an adequate peripheral iridectomy, though vitreous herniation through an iridectomy may also result in failure, if a trabeculectomy is performed on an aphakic eye. Elevated resistance at the level of the scleral flap may be due to healing of the actual flap, but is more commonly due to

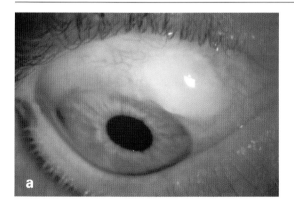 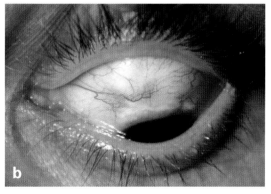

Figure 3.3 The bleb resulting from a limbus-based conjunctival flap (a) tends to develop a more focal morophology and is located closer to the limbus than that resulting from the fornix-based flap trabeculectomy (b).

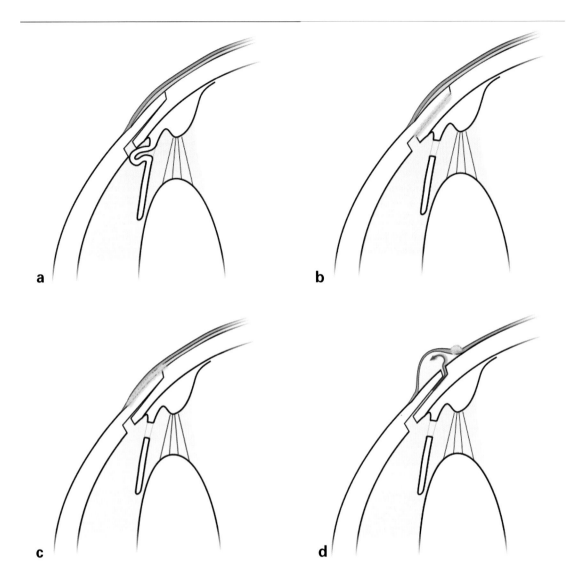

Figure 3.4 Filtration failure may occur at one or more of the following four sites: (a) the sclerostomy may become obstructed by iris or vitreous within the anterior chamber; (b) healing of the scleral flap may obstruct outflow; (c) episcleral fibrosis at the external aperture of the sclerostomy prevents aqueous entering the subconjunctival space; and (d) aqueous entering the subconjunctival space becomes trapped within a bleb that is encapsulated in scar tissue (bleb encystment).

episcleral fibrosis which may also obliterate the subconjunctival space over the flap preventing bleb formation. Finally, encystment of the bleb may occur in a patient with normal scleral flap function due to peripheral subconjunctival scarring which delimits the bleb, prevents aqueous

absorption and elevates internal bleb pressure to that of the anterior chamber.

The common factor in most cases of filtration failure is excessive scarring in the subconjunctival space (see Figure 3.4c,d) and this may be reduced using antiscarring agents such as 5-fluorouracil

(5-FU) and MMC (Figure 3.5). These two cytotoxic agents appear to act at least partially via induction of apoptosis.

MMC is an antibiotic derived from the fungus *Streptomyces caespitosus* and can act as an alkylating agent preventing DNA synthesis. MMC has the advantage of a prolonged effect from a single intraoperative dose. In vivo, MMC produces permanent inhibition of fibroblast division after a 5-minute exposure, whereas inhibition after 5-FU exposure is temporary. 5-FU is consequently less effective in preventing subconjunctival scarring than MMC and traditionally has been given as multiple postoperative subconjunctival injections, although a significant effect has also been demonstrated using a single intraoperative dose.

The Fluorouracil Filtering Surgery study demonstrated that with multiple postoperative injections of 5-FU, less than 50% of high-risk trabeculectomies were still functioning successfully at 5 years. Mitomycin appears to result in better longevity of trabeculectomy function in patients at a high risk of failure with the convenience of a single intraoperative dose. Although there are few comparative studies, there exists a large body of clinical experience and some published clinical series, confirming the expected superior potency of MMC over 5-FU

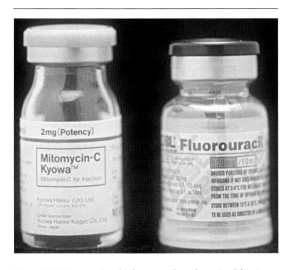

Figure 3.5 Mitomycin C and 5-fluorouracil are the antiproliferative agents commonly used in clinical practice.

in trabeculectomies at a high risk of failure. The difference is less clear-cut in lower risk cases, where arguably the use of 5-FU might be more appropriate for safety reasons. As MMC is more potent than 5-FU, the risks associated with its use are also higher. These include postoperative hypotony and bleb-related infection.

INDICATIONS FOR ANTIMETABOLITE USE

MMC is used in the cases at highest risk of failure or those in which a low target IOP range is deemed to be necessary. 5-FU is used in low and intermediate risk cases although practice varies. Some surgeons do not use antiproliferatives in cases without risk factors for failure.

Because of the findings on the benefits of low target IOPs from the Advanced Glaucoma Intervention Study (AGIS), many ophthalmologists consider MMC appropriate in patients who have a lower risk of trabeculectomy failure but require low target IOPs.

The improved efficacy of glaucoma medications in the late 1990s has resulted in an overall decrease in the total numbers of trabeculectomies performed. This has not been matched in the author's institution by any change in the annual number of mitomycin trabeculectomies. It appears that improvements in medical therapy have reduced the numbers of lower risk trabeculectomies without significantly affecting the numbers of higher risk cases. As a result, there has been a shift in the trabeculectomy case mix towards a higher risk, more subspecialized, group. Currently over 50% of primary trabeculectomies in the USA are performed with MMC (Rich Parrish, MD, 2002 Survey of the American Glaucoma Society personal communication).

HOW TO APPLY ANTIMETABOLITES

5-FLUOROURACIL

5-FU may be given intraoperatively on a sponge or via a series of postoperative injections. Postoperative injections may be given into the lower or upper fornices but different volumes and concentrations are used according to the exact injection site. A large volume (1 ml) of a low concentration (5 mg/ml) to the lower fornix allows sufficient spread to influence the superior conjunctiva without risking an intraocular injection of 5-FU, but probably delivers a lower dose to the target site than a small volume (0.1 ml) of a higher concentration (50 mg/ml) containing the same amount of drug (5 mg) and injected via the upper fornix, close to the target site. Injection of either concentration requires good topical anesthesia with tetracaine, especially when injecting the 50 mg/ml concentration which has a very high pH and is extremely irritating. An advantage of the higher concentration and smaller volume may be the reduced area of contact with consequently a lower incidence of corneal epitheliopathy.

A single intraoperative exposure to 5-FU delivers a lower dose than a series of postoperative injections but appears to have comparable efficacy in vitro. A single dose is clearly more convenient and also results in less corneal epitheliopathy.

MITOMYCIN C

MMC is given as a single intraoperative application usually on one or more sponges. The exposure concentration ranges from 0.1 to 0.5 mg/ml and the duration of application ranges from 1 to 5 minutes. Three minutes appear to provide optimal scleral uptake whereas longer durations of exposure are more likely to result in hypotony. Similarly the use of concentrations in the region of 0.2 mg/ml provide a good balance between efficacy and hypotony, although for very high failure risk cases, concentrations of 0.4–0.5 mg/ml may be necessary. In the higher doses, MMC has been shown to cause hypotony in the absence of external drainage, presumably from mild ciliary epithelial necrosis.

Area and method of MMC applicaton: MMC is generally applied on a sponge under conjunctiva/Tenon's before or after scleral flap dissection. The target cells of MMC application are the fibroblasts of Tenon's capsule and episclera that cause trabeculectomy failure as outlined in Figure 3.4.

Failure primarily due to healing of the scleral flap is less common. Application of MMC prior to scleral dissection should therefore treat the primary target tissue with a reduced risk of intraocular exposure. In cases where a large surface area scleral flap is required, a larger area of contact for scleral healing results and the argument for subscleral MMC application is stronger. On the other hand, a smaller surface area flap may only warrant episcleral application. The author's preferred technique is to apply mitomycin C prior to scleral dissection and to make a relatively broad short scleral flap. Either way it is preferable not to apply MMC after the anterior chamber has been opened.

While the type of conjunctival flap appears to influence the type of bleb produced, as discussed above, the method of application of MMC seems also to be important. A wide area of application is more likely to produce a diffuse bleb with less thinning of the bleb roof. This can be achieved using multiple small sponges soaked in mitomycin C over a wide area posterior to the anticipated site of the scleral flap site (Figure 3.6). Polyvinyl alcohol sponges, such as corneal light shields (Merocel, see above), have a low profile, tend not to fragment and lend themselves well to the delivery of MMC.

As discussed previously, the site of exposure is also important. While inferiorly placed trabeculectomies are clearly at a higher risk of late infection, significant bleb dysesthesia may also be induced if the bleb forms in the interpalpebral space (Figure 3.7). Exposure of nasal and temporal interpalpebral conjunctiva to MMC should therefore be avoided by keeping the area of MMC exposure as close as possible to the 12 o'clock position.

PRECAUTIONS WHEN USING ANTIMETABOLITES

A number of countries have specific regulations or guidelines relating to the handling of these agents. These are generally designed to protect both the patient and the operating room staff from these extremely toxic drugs. In general such guidelines specify that at minimum, a separate sterile work area should be used for mixing cytotoxic agents and staff handling these drugs should wear protective glasses and disposable gloves. Care must be taken when mixing cytotoxic agents so as not to cause

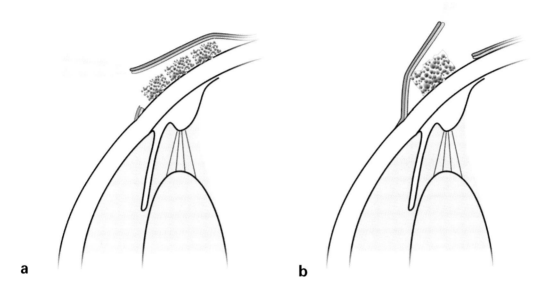

Figure 3.6 The fornix-based flap (a) lends itself to a wide area of application of MMC on multiple sponges. Alternatively a limbus-based flap can be used with the more traditional single large sponge application of MMC (b).

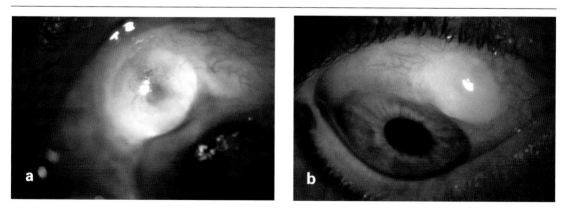

Figure 3.7 (a,b) The ideal bleb is positioned at 12 o'clock. Nasal and temporal blebs may not be fully covered by the eyelid and may result in dysesthetic ocular surface symptoms.

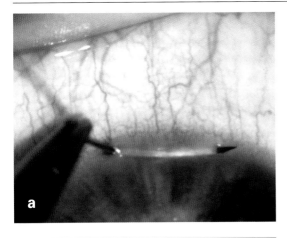

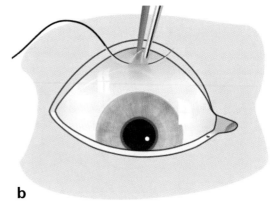

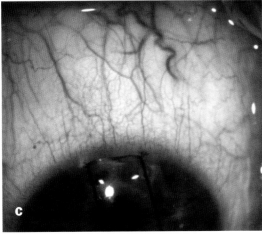

Figure 3.8 A peripheral corneal traction suture (a) gives good control of the globe during surgery without the hazards of bleeding, ptosis and superior rectus trauma that result from a superior rectus suture (b). Good superior conjunctival exposure is achieved with a peripheral corneal traction suture close to the 12 o'clock limbus, without compromising surgical access (c).

backspray or aerosol formation and ideally these procedures should be performed in a laminar flow cabinet.

During the application of MMC, care should be taken to localize the area of exposure to the area intended so that other tissues are not inadvertently treated. Ideally the cut conjunctival edge should be protected from exposure as much as possible to minimize the risk of delayed healing of the conjunctival flap. After the use of MMC, the area of application is irrigated thoroughly, to terminate tissue exposure to the agent. Care must also be taken to dispose of these agents in a manner that prevents unnecessary risk to other staff and the environment.

SURGICAL TECHNIQUE – STEP-BY-STEP

After adequate anesthesia, the eye is initially prepared and draped as appropriate for any intraocular procedure. When administering local anesthesia it is worth using a long-acting agent such as bupivacaine as well as lidocaine to ensure a sufficient duration of action. Topical anesthesia is less satisfactory for filtration surgery than for phacoemulsification, especially where antiproliferative application and releasable sutures are likely to prolong the procedure. A corneal light shield or an equivalent sponge should be placed on the cornea from the start of the procedure to protect the retina

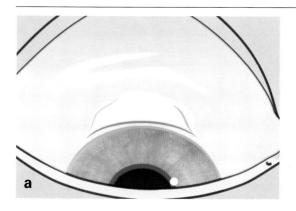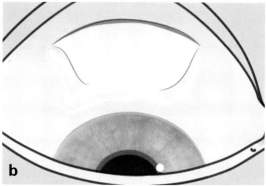

Figure 3.9 The initial conjunctival incision is made circumferential and adjacent to the limbus for the fornix-based conjunctival flap (a) and approximately 6 mm posterior to the limbus for the limbus-based conjunctival flap (b). With the fornix-based flap (a), Tenon's incision is made through Tenon's insertion and the two layers are reflected together. With the limbus-based flap, the conjunctiva should be reflected forwards and Tenon's incised anterior to the insertion of superior rectus to avoid muscle trauma and bleeding (b).

from photic damage, especially in eyes with advanced glaucoma.

TRACTION SUTURE

A 7-0 silk traction suture on a spatulated needle is anchored in the peripheral cornea at 12 o'clock (Figure 3.8). This allows good control of globe position, especially when applying antiproliferative agents, without the added problems associated with a superior rectus suture, i.e. subconjunctival bleeding, conjunctival button hole, and postoperative ptosis. The corneal traction suture is more hazardous to insert in the patient with peripheral corneal thinning or a corneal extracapsular cataract wound. However, there are few instances in which it is not possible to insert such a suture safely and in such cases, an inferior corneal traction suture or parallel traction sutures through nasal and temporal limbus may be preferable to a superior rectus suture.

CONJUNCTIVAL DISSECTION

Construction of a fornix-based conjunctival flap simply requires a peritomy at the limbus through approximately 2 clock hours usually from 11 to 1 o'clock without a radial relaxing incision (Figure 3.9). Tenon's incision is then made through Tenon's insertion and the two layers reflected together. The posterior application of MMC is then facilitated by a posterior sub-Tenon's dissection to open up the subconjunctival space on either side of the superior rectus muscle (Figure 3.10). Care should be taken to avoid trauma to the muscle to preserve hemostasis.

A limbus-based flap is made via a horizontal incision in the conjunctiva at least 6 mm posterior to the limbus. Tenon's capsule is incised anterior to the insertion of superior rectus to avoid muscle trauma and bleeding.

ANTI-METABOLITE APPLICATION

It is important to achieve good hemostasis prior to antimetabolite application. In vitro fetal calf serum inhibits the induction of apoptosis by MMC and one might expect blood in the operative site to have the same effect. The author's preference is to use an eraser-style cautery (Figure 3.11).

After hemostasis is achieved, antimetabolites are applied, using for example small nonfragmenting sponges such as halved corneal light shields as previously discussed (Figure 3.12). After the sponges have been removed, the area of exposure is washed thoroughly with approximately 20 ml of a phsyiological saline solution such as Aqsia (Chauvin).

PARACENTESIS

An anterior chamber paracentesis is ideally performed after removal of 5-FU or MMC to minimize

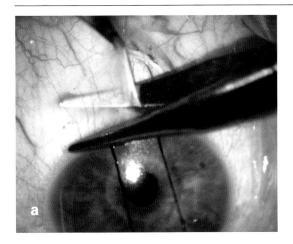

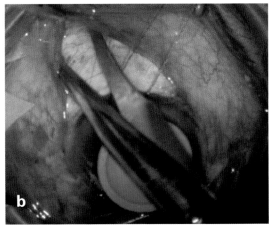

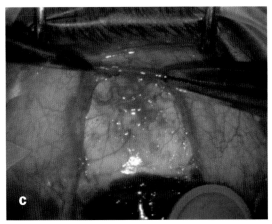

Figure 3.10 The fornix-based conjunctival flap incision (a), posterior dissection to one side of superior rectus (b), the anterior margin of superior rectus just visible beneath the conjunctival edge after dissection (c).

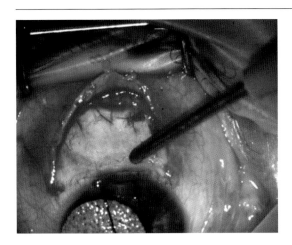

Figure 3.11 Good hemostasis is essential prior to antiproliferative application. The advantage of an eraser cautery becomes more apparent when fashioning the scleral flap. An eraser with a fine point can be used to target small bleeding points in the flap with minimal flap shrinkage.

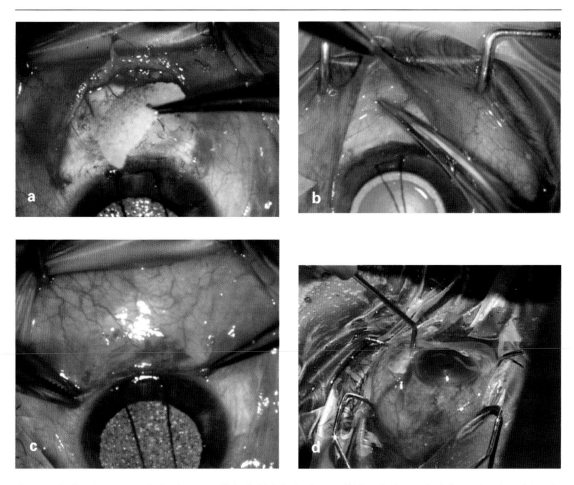

Figure 3.12 (a–d) Mitomycin C applied on four corneal light shields halved and inserted high under the superior bulbar conjunctiva and Tenon's on either side of the superior rectus. Following application MMC exposure is terminated by irrigation with a large volume (e.g. 20 ml) of Ringer's solution.

the risk of intraocular exposure, but is most easily performed when the eye is still firm (Figure 3.13).

It is perhaps best performed prior to dissection of the scleral flap, so as not to be forgotten. The same is true of the corneal grooves if releasable sutures are planned (Figure 3.14). Although a paracentesis is relatively easy to perform, it is worth taking care to ensure that no trauma to the lens or iris occurs while making a paracentesis. This is especially true in phakic eyes with shallow anterior chambers. The entry site should be self-sealing even in the event of postoperative hypotony. Ideally, the paracentesis should be sited

in temporal cornea to facilitate postoperative access at the slit-lamp.

An effective paracentesis can be made with a 23–25-gauge needle or blade. The larger the instrument, the higher the risk of lens trauma and the longer the tunnel required for a self-sealing wound. The instrument used to make the paracentesis, whether blade or needle, should be introduced into the anterior chamber in a plane parallel to the iris surface. In cases with very shallow anterior chambers, a paracentesis can be performed obliquely rather than radially in the peripheral cornea, minimizing the risk of perforating lens capsule.

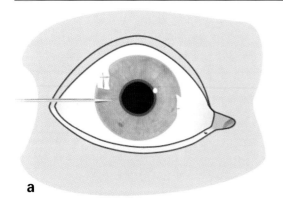

a

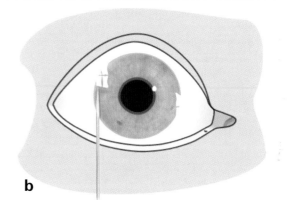

b

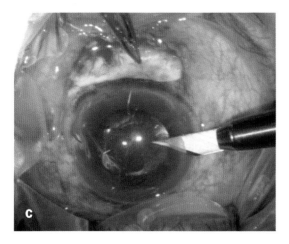

c

Figure 3.13 (a,b) A radial paracentesis can be made using a hypodermic needle or fine blade. In phakic eyes, or cases with very shallow anterior chambers it is worth considering a tangential or oblique entry in order to avoid lens trauma. (c) Paracentesis in a small pseudophakic eye using a feather blade.

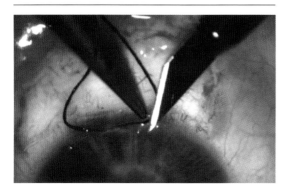

Figure 3.14 If releasable scleral flap sutures are to be buried in the peripheral cornea, it is easier to prepare the grooves prior to fashioning the scleral flap while the eye is still firm.

THE SCLERAL FLAP

Various shapes of scleral flap have been described. Irrespective of the shape, a few general principles are important.

The basic requirement for a scleral flap is to cover sufficiently the sclerostomy to provide some resistance to outflow. Ideally, the flap should be thick enough so that it can be sutured tightly without risk of button-holing and it should extend sufficiently far posteriorly so that it is possible to achieve a watertight seal if necessary. Traditionally the sides of the flap have been cut right up to the limbus. While this is unnecessary in most cases, it is usually necessary to open the sides to around 1 mm from the limbus to prevent a self-sealing trabeculectomy.

Area and thickness: While adequate coverage of the sclerostomy site is paramount, flap dimensions in excess of 2 mm from the sclerostomy on any side are probably excessive and increases the surface area for healing. The larger the flap surface area, the greater the likelihood of healing. If a large surface area flap is deemed to be necessary, then it may be necessary to expose the undersurface of the flap to MMC to limit healing. Likewise, a thin flap, while ideal for filtration, is more susceptible to shrinkage with cautery, necrosis from the long-term effects of MMC, and more difficult to close when suturing.

If the primary aim is to produce posterior drainage of aqueous, then the type of flap that can best achieve that aim will be more broad than long. In other words, the distance from the posterior edge of the sclerostomy to the posterior edge of the flap should be less than the distance from the nasal and temporal edges of the sclerostomy to their respective flap edges. The line of least resistance to

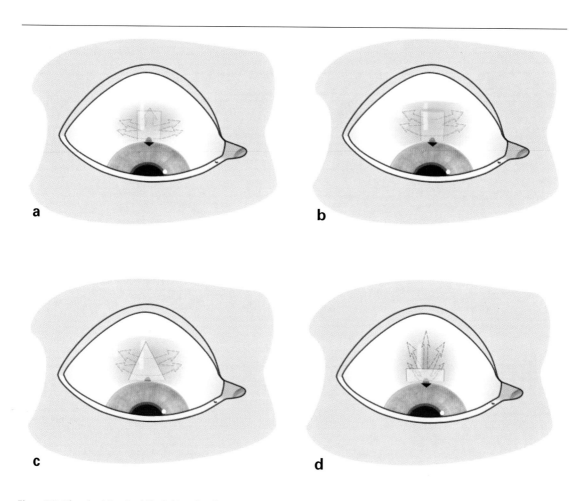

a

b

c

d

Figure 3.15 The scleral flap should be fashioned so that the line of least resistance to aqueous flow is away from the limbus. A flap with a long anterior–posterior dimension (a) results in more lateral than posterior flow of aqueous. Lack of posterior flow allows the posterior margin of the flap to heal (b) further increasing the degree of lateral flow. A triangular flap encourages more posterior flow (c), but still less than a broad flap with a short anterior–posterior diameter (d).

aqueous flow will then be backwards so that posterior drainage is achieved (Figure 3.15).

Fashioning the flap: In the author's practice the scleral flap is made in a fashion analogous to that of the scleral tunnel previously used for non-corneal phacoemulsification. A 4 mm straight cut is made to approximately 60% scleral depth, 2 mm posterior and tangential to the superior limbus. A lamellar tunnel is fashioned by advancing a crescent knife in the same plane until it enters the peripheral cornea (Figure 3.16). The anterior chamber is then entered

with a slit knife (keratome) and the sides of the flap are cut with the same blade.

The more traditional alternative is to outline all three flap edges by making a groove to 60% scleral depth with a blade and fashioning a flap by lamellar dissection up to the limbus with a blade. At that point the anterior chamber is entered with a blade.

It is necessary to open the sides of the scleral flap right up to the limbus if the sclerostomy will be created by cutting a block (see below). If a punch is to be used, the sides can be opened to approximately

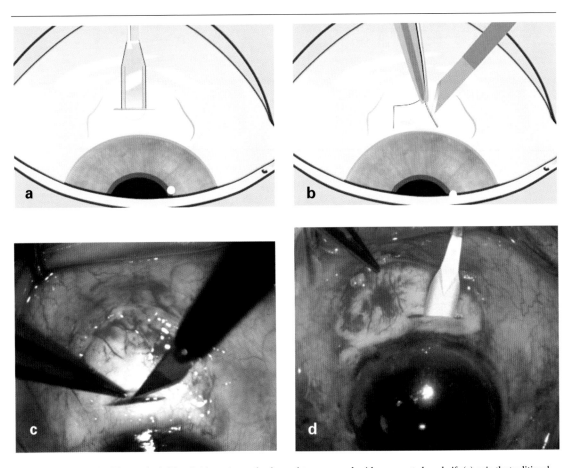

Figure 3.16 (a–h) A scleral flap can be fashioned either using a scleral tunnel-type approach with a crescent phaco knife (a) or in the traditional fashion (b). Using the scleral tunnel-style approach, a slit knife (keratome) can be used to enter the anterior chamber. As a result the sides of the scleral flap are not opened to the limbus and the likelihood of leakage from the anterior margins of the sides of the flap is reduced.

1 mm posterior to the limbus. Incomplete opening of the sides of the flap reduces the risk of postoperative bleb leakage, but also occasionally can result in a self-sealing trabeculectomy.

SCLEROSTOMY

The sclerostomy is something of a misnomer as the internal opening is normally in the peripheral cornea rather than the sclera. There are two ways of fashioning a sclerostomy. The first is to use a Descemet's punch, such as the Kelly or Luntz-Dodick (Figure 3.17a,b). If a punch is not available or a trabecular meshwork specimen is desired for histologic examination, then a trabeculectomy block can be excised using a fine blade. In the traditional Cairn's type trabeculectomy, a 3 × 1 mm block is excised (Figure 3.17c). To do this, the scleral flap must be opened to the limbus. The punch offers a number of advantages over a block when fashioning a sclerostomy. It is quick, requires less skill, and can be done easily without opening the flap fully, or even at all in some cases where the flap is short (Figure 3.18).

Although the Watson style trabeculectomy involved a true sclerectomy, most trabeculectomies today avoid crossing the limbus into sclera because it is not necessary for drainage and may be associated with excessive bleeding (Figure 3.19).

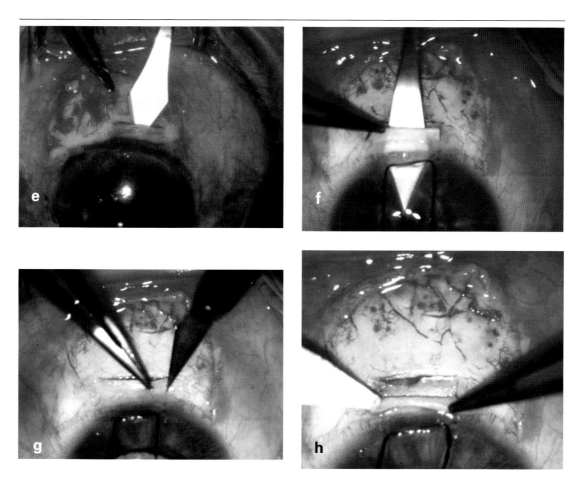

Figure 3.16 (a–h) continued (e,f) entering anterior chamber with blade, (g) opening up the sites of the scleral flap, (h) scleral flap.

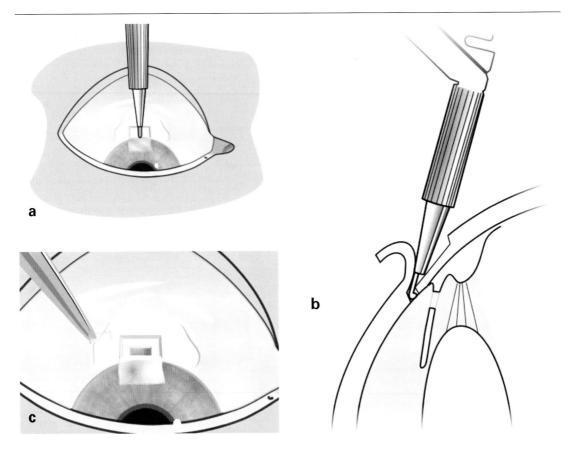

Figure 3.17 If the scleral flap is not opened fully, then a punch is required to perform the sclerostomy (a,b). The alternative method is to cut a block with a blade and this method is essential if trabecular tissue is required for histologic examination (c).

PERIPHERAL IRIDECTOMY

As the peripheral iris lies in close proximity to a correctly placed sclerostomy in all but the deepest of anterior chambers, a peripheral iridectomy is essential to prevent obstruction of the sclerostomy. A peripheral iridectomy is fashioned by lifting the scleral flap, at which point the peripheral iris will often prolapse through the sclerostomy. A small portion of iris is then excised using either De Wecker's or Vannas scissors (Figure 3.20).

Care must be taken to ensure that the iridectomy is full-thickness and that it is of an appropriate size. Occasionally it may be appropriate to first constrict a dilated pupil in order to avoid making an excessively large peripheral iridectomy by injecting a small amount of acetylcholine chloride (Miochol). This scenario can also be avoided in most cases by instilling a drop of 1% pilocarpine preoperatively. If the pupil is constricted and does not prolapse easily, fine grooved or toothed forceps may be required to help the iris prolapse through the sclerostomy. Care must be taken in this situation to avoid lens trauma.

After fashioning the peripheral iridectomy and prior to scleral flap closure, injection of BSS via the paracentesis should result in free flow of aqueous through a well-positioned sclerostomy. If it does not, there will be no postoperative drainage. A self-sealing sclerostomy is most likely to result from a phaco-type scleral tunnel which has not been

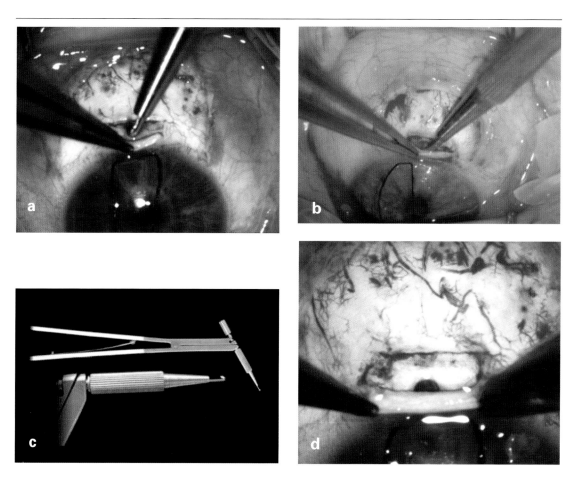

Figure 3.18 (a–d) A sclerostomy made with a punch. The punch illustrated is the Luntz-Dodick (Katena).

opened sufficiently at the sides, or when a punch is used to fashion a trabeculectomy from a slit-knife incision that is too anterior in the peripheral cornea (see Figure 3.19).

CLOSURE OF THE SCLERAL FLAP

In general, if an antimetabolite is used, the scleral flap must be tightly sutured to prevent hypotony. As the normal rate of aqueous production is in the order of 2 μl/minute, any visible drainage is likely to exceed that figure. This is less of a problem in eyes that have not been exposed to an antimetabolite as the normal healing response will often prevent excessive early outflow.

A tight-suturing technique can result in a high postoperative IOP, a situation that can be remedied by bleb massage at the slit-lamp to establish filtration and lower the IOP to the desired target range. This degree of postoperative control can be enhanced by using sutures which can either be cut by argon laser or removed at the slit-lamp when required.

Fixed sutures: 10-0 nylon fixed interrupted sutures have traditionally been used to close the scleral flap. These have the advantage of stability in that they are highly unlikely to unravel postoperatively. If lowering of the IOP is required postoperatively

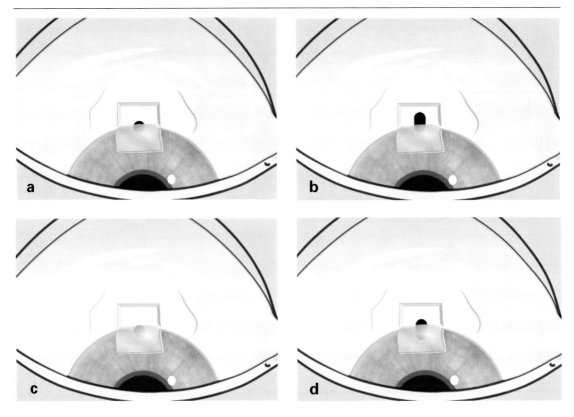

Figure 3.19 Importance of sclerostomy position: (a) a correctly-fashioned punch sclerostomy can drain freely when the flap is unsutured but does not extend posteriorly into sclera; (b) if the sclerostomy does extend posteriorly into sclera unnecessary excessive bleeding may be encountered; (c) if the initial anterior chamber entry site is anteriorly positioned, care must be taken not to create a self-sealing trabeculectomy; in which case (d) several bites may be required with the punch to produce an adequate sclerostomy.

then these sutures can be cut with an Argon laser to increase filtration.

Releasable sutures: There are a number of methods of tying releasable sutures. The method described here is that used in the author's institution (Figures 3.21 and 3.22). The salient features of this type of suture are:

- The slip knot has four throws. Four throws ensures stability of the knot without preventing release.
- There is a loop buried in a shallow groove in the peripheral cornea. This can be easily released from its corneal site and then pulled with a pair of plain forceps to release the entire suture. The

buried loop ensures that it can be left in situ in the longer term if clinically indicated, without exposing the patient to an unnecessary risk of infection.

- There is a short subconjunctival loop. A long subconjunctival loop easily becomes embedded in subconjunctival scar tissue. The slip knot with four throws ensures sufficient stability for the subconjunctival loop to be left short and hence easy to remove postoperatively.

When closure of the scleral flap is complete, it is important to test the integrity of the wound by injecting BSS into the anterior chamber via a paracentesis to ensure that no more than a slow ooze of drainage can be detected. If excessive drainage is

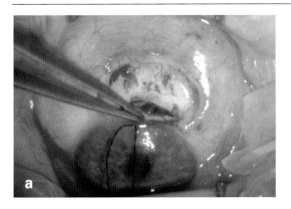

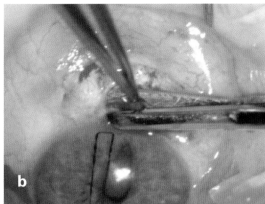

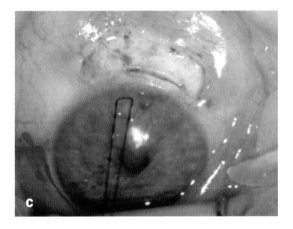

Figure 3.20 (a–c) A peripheral iridotomy is essential except in some pseudophakic eyes with deep anterior chambers.

visualized, the scleral sutures can be tightened or additional sutures added. It is less logical to inject BSS after conjunctival closure is complete, when no adjustment of scleral tension is possible (Figure 3.23).

CONJUNCTIVAL CLOSURE

Closure of a fornix-based flap requires greater attention to detail than a limbus-based flap for a number of reasons. First, loose closure may permit aqueous leakage in the early postoperative period. After exposure to MMC, delayed healing may result and the leak may persist for some time. As a result, the tissue separation between the conjunctiva and sclera which is necessary to establish a satisfactory bleb does not occur. When the leak eventually heals, the trabeculectomy may have failed. Secondly, loose suturing of a fornix-based flap may

result in postoperative conjunctival recession to such an extent that the limbal conjunctiva lies posterior to the scleral flap. This may happen even in patients with adequate conjunctiva that is not under tension in the operating room. In this situation, resuturing of the conjunctiva is mandatory.

There are three principles of suturing a fornix-based flap: (i) to stretch the limbal edge of the conjunctiva by closing the extremities of the flap as if there were relaxing incisions on each side; (ii) to close these imaginary relaxing incisions with a pursestring or small locked running suture to ensure no gaps develop; and (iii) at least one central mattress suture at the limbal edge is essential to prevent conjunctival recession. The author's preference is to use 10-0 nylon for conjunctival closure as it is less inflammatory than Vicryl. 8-0 or 10-0 Vicryl may be used, but both are

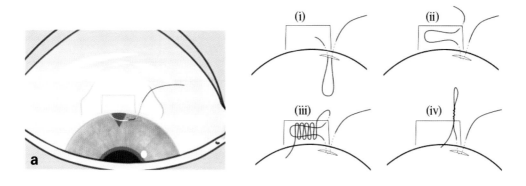

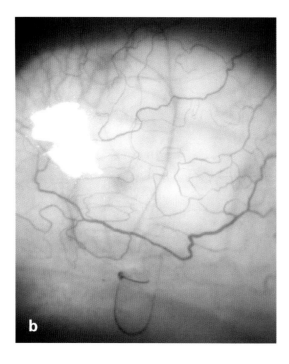

Figure 3.21 (a,b) Releasable sutures permit the flexibility of opening the flap manually if massage is insufficient to reduce a high postoperative pressure. Four throws on the knot (iii) ensure stability of the knot, while a short loop prevents the suture material becoming embedded in Tenon's and obstructing later removal. A shallow peripheral corneal groove is essential so that the corneal portion of the suture can be buried. Burying the corneal portion allows the surgeon the flexibility of leaving the suture in place permanently should removal be undesirable.

more inflammatory, and in the author's experience, neither absorbs sufficiently quickly enough to not require physical removal at the slit-lamp (usually 2–3 weeks after surgery).

When suturing is complete, it is possible to test the integrity of the conjunctival closure for a leak, by injecting viscoelastic such as Healon or Provisc under the conjunctiva to inflate the bleb artificially and then to look for gaps in the conjunctival wound (Figure 3.24). Extra sutures can then be applied as

required. This technique gives the added advantage of some mechanical separation of the conjunctiva from the sclera in the early postoperative period which may help prevent adherence of these two tissues and provide a subconjunctival area for bleb formation when drainage is established later.

POSTOPERATIVE CARE

To achieve a high success rate from filtration surgery, especially in more complex cases, intensive

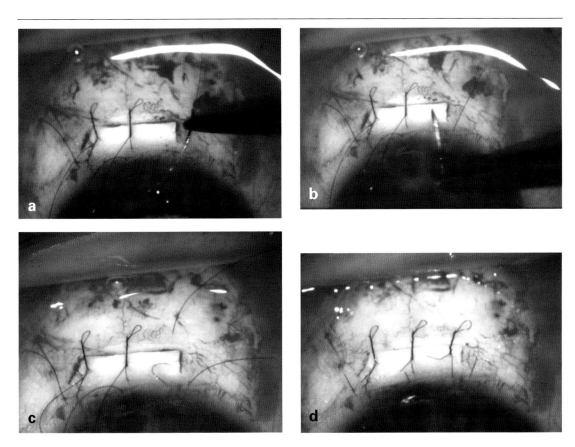

Figure 3.22 (a–d) This illustration demonstrates how a flap can be sutured tightly exclusively with releasable sutures. The stability of the sutures and integrity of the scleral flap should be tested at this stage by injecting balanced salt solution into the anterior chamber via the paracentesis and observing the presence or absence of drainage.

postoperative care is almost as important as careful intraoperative technique. Good postoperative care often involves more intensive topical cortico-steroids than after cataract surgery, regular bleb massage, suture removal or laser suture lysis, and subconjunctival 5-FU injections if underdrainage occurs.

As a result of the tight scleral suturing technique described above, the IOP may be high on the first postoperative day. Gentle bleb massage at the slit lamp will usually initiate drainage and is carried out by depressing the patient's upper lid after instillation of local anesthetic such as benoxinate or proxymeta-caine. The appearance of a bleb and a measurable reduction in IOP should be confirmed by recheck-ing the eye after a further 20 minutes. Removal of

releasable sutures and laser suture lysis are generally not performed in the first postoperative week in MMC trabeculectomies because of the risk of profound hypotony from ensuing overdrainage. However, after 2–4 postoperative weeks, a high IOP unresponsive or poorly responsive to bleb massage may well respond to suture release.

MANAGEMENT OF INTRAOPERATIVE HAZARDS AND POSTOPERATIVE COMPLICATIONS

INTRAOPERATIVE HAZARDS

The trabeculectomy procedure itself may be sur-gically challenging in certain eyes, especially small hypermetropic eyes. An eye with a shallow anterior

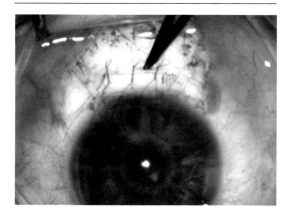

Figure 3.23 In high risk cases it is desirable to adjust suture tension so that no spontaneous drainage occurs when the anterior chamber is irrigated with BSS, but that drainage is easily established by depressing the posterior lip (analogous to postoperative massage).

chamber has less space to accommodate any intraocular instrumentation, and has a greater risk of intraoperative shallowing and of lens trauma from instrumentation within the eye. It is worth considering the use of a viscoelastic agent to maintain the anterior chamber and applying topical 1% atropine at the end of the procedure in these patients.

An oblique paracentesis, almost tangential with the limbus, rather than radial is worth considering in these higher risk eyes (see Figure 3.13). The ante-

rior chamber, if required, can then be re-formed with reduced risk of trauma to the crystalline lens.

Intraoperative hazards that may be encountered include hyphema, anterior chamber shallowing, lens trauma, vitreous presentation, and iris prolapse.

Hyphema: This is a relatively common complication a of trabeculectomy, and bleeding may occur either from the scleral wound or the iris root. Bleeding from the scleral flap can be controlled using diathermy. Bleeding from the sclerostomy can be avoided by placing the sclerostomy in the peripheral cornea rather than in the sclera. Bleeding from the iris root is avoided by not tearing or traumatizing the iris root when creating the peripheral iridectomy. Excessive hemorrhage from the iris or sclerostomy site is best controlled by closing the sclerostomy tightly and increasing the IOP, since they are both difficult to stop with diathermy.

Anterior chamber shallowing: During the filtration procedure, after the sclerostomy has been fashioned, and while the scleral flap is still open, the filtration site is completely unguarded, unless scleral flap sutures have been preplaced. Anterior chamber shallowing is most likely to occur at this point. The tendency to shallow can be prevented by minimizing forward pressure on the iris-lens diaphragm. This is achieved by ensuring that there is no pres-

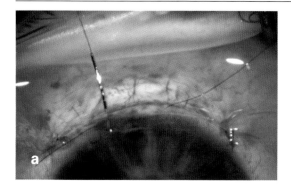
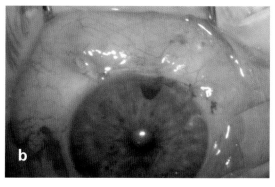

Figure 3.24 (a,b) A fornix-based conjunctival flap may recess postoperatively and therefore one or more central mattress sutures are required to anchor the conjunctiva at the limbus. Similarly, to prevent postoperative leakage it is important to close the conjunctiva tightly at the lateral margins of the wound (a). The integrity of the conjunctival closure can be demonstrated by injected viscoelastic under the edge of the conjunctiva to inflate the bleb (a). Any defects in suturing then become apparent as gaping of the conjunctival wound.

sure on the globe from the eyelid speculum. In cases deemed to be at especially high risk of shallowing, posterior vitreous pressure can be reduced by general anesthesia rather than local anesthesia.

Intracameral injection of viscoelastic such as Healon or Provisc can help reduce the tendency for the anterior chamber to shallow. The duration of this *unguarded* period can be minimized with pre-placed scleral flap sutures which can immediately be tightened after the peripheral iridectomy has been made. After the scleral sutures have been tightened, further shallowing will only occur if the scleral flap or suturing technique is inadequate to maintain the anterior chamber, or there is increased posterior chamber pressure, such as a suprachoroidal hemorrhage.

Lens trauma: Even an uncomplicated trabeculectomy results in an increased rate of cataract formation. The formation of cataracts can be exacerbated intraoperatively by inadvertent lens trauma. Lens trauma may occur from a blade used to fashion the paracentesis or to create the iridectomy or scleral incision. The risk of lens trauma is greatest when operating on a phakic eye in which the anterior chamber is already shallow. Gentle pressure posterior to the sclerostomy site may help the iris prolapse out and allow the surgeon to grasp the iris without reaching into the anterior chamber.

Vitreous presentation: This may occur not only in aphakic but also in pseudophakic and occasionally, even in phakic eyes. It usually occurs through a peripheral iridectomy just after it has been made. This may occur because of pre-existing zonular disruption from prior trauma, or a pseudoexfoliation, or because of inadvertent cutting of the zonule during the iridectomy. An anterior vitrectomy is essential to prevent vitreous from blocking the trabeculectomy.

POSTOPERATIVE COMPLICATIONS

Certain eyes are predisposed to develop postoperative hypotony after a trabeculectomy.

Eyes of uveitic patients, younger patients, and high myopes have a greater risk of ocular hypotony after filtration surgery. Tight closure of the scleral

flap is important in myopes who tend to have greater scleral elasticity and consequently a greater tendency to develop hypotony maculopathy. Aphakic eyes have a greater risk of postoperative suprachoroidal hemorrhages and vitreous presentation. Hypermetropic eyes are at increased risk of postoperative anterior chamber shallowing and malignant glaucoma.

Early postoperative bleb leakage predisposes to bleb failure and also causes ocular hypotony. This is because aqueous drainage in the first few postoperative weeks plays an important role in establishing the boundaries of the mature bleb by mechanically separating the conjunctiva and Tenon's capsule from the sclera and hence helping to prevent healing of the subconjunctival space. If the draining aqueous simply leaks away, it does not perform this necessary role. In addition, there is an increased risk of infection. The simplest way to reduce early leakage is to allow healing to accelerate by reducing the intensity of postoperative topical steroids. This may be aided by tamponade with a bandage contact lens. Sometimes the author also uses aqueous suppressants. As soon as the leak is healed, the intensity of topical steroid administration can be increased again as required. If leakage is due to conjunctival recession over the scleral flap, then surgical intervention to repair the conjunctiva is indicated.

Early postoperative hypotony may be due to overdrainage and its management depends on the amount of hypotony. Hypotony maculopathy requires aggressive intervention because vision is threatened. If the anterior chamber remains formed and the best-corrected pin hole acuity is 20/40 or better, conservative management is not unreasonable. However, if there is a shallow or flat anterior chamber and severe hypotony maculopathy, surgical intervention may be required to prevent permanent visual loss.

Conservative management of postoperative hypotony involves reduction or withdrawal of postoperative topical steroids, and bleb tamponade with a large therapeutic contact lens or Simmon's shell. The aim of surgical intervention is to increase scleral resistance and the first step should be to resuture the scleral flap more tightly. If this cannot be achieved, then it is worth considering patching the sclerostomy with autologous Tenon's capsule or donor tissue, such as donor sclera or pericardium.

A less common cause of hypotony is the decreased production of aqueous which may occur because of ciliary body dysfunction. This is seen in patients who are uveitic, who have had previous cyclophotocoagulation, or who have been exposed to heavy doses of MMC, or are young. The diagnosis of ciliary body underproduction as a cause of ocular hypotony in patients is a difficult clinical task, especially if there is visible external drainage. In patients with no visible external drainage and no wound leaks, the diagnosis of ciliary body underproduction is easier.

Patients with advanced glaucoma and preoperative split fixation on visual field testing, have a significant risk of wipeout of the remaining visual field after filtration surgery. In patients with advanced glaucoma but good central vision, the author will not perform intraocular surgery without a preoperative 10-2 central visual field to clarify the threat to fixation. In these cases it may be worth boosting topical steroid administration to stimulate aqueous flow. In addition, intraocular injection of viscoelastic or even perfluoropropane or sulfur hexafluoride gas in aphakes may help keep the chamber formed and the eye pressure elevated until aqueous production improves.

CONCLUSION

Trabeculectomies are deceptively simple procedures that can be quite challenging to have work successfully, since the natural tendency is for the eye to heal the sclerostomy. In fact, it is quite amazing how successful they can be. Attention to detail, pre-, intra-, and postoperatively, can make a big difference to the success of the operation.

ACKNOWLEDGEMENTS

All line drawings are the work of Mr Alan Lacey of Moorfields Eye Hospital and are reproduced with his kind permission.

FURTHER READING

AGIS investigators. The advanced glaucoma intervention study, 8: risk of cataract formation after trabeculectomy. Arch Ophthalmol 2001; 119: 1771–9.

AGIS investigators. The advanced glaucoma intervention study (AGIS): 7. The relationship between control of intraocular pressure and visual field deterioration. The AGIS investigators. Am J Ophthalmol 2000; 130: 429–40.

Budenz DL, Hoffman K, Zacchei A. Glaucoma filtering bleb dysesthesia. Am J Ophthalmol 2001; 131: 626–30.

Caronia RM, Liebmann JM, Friedman R, Cohen H, Ritch R. Trabeculectomy at the inferior limbus. Arch Ophthalmol 1996; 114: 387–91.

Chen PP, Yamamoto T, Sawada A, Parrish RK, Kitazawa Y. Use of antifibrosis agents and glaucoma drainage devices in the American and Japanese Glaucoma Societies. J Glaucoma 1997; 6: 192–6.

Chen PP, Weaver YK, Budenz DL, Feuer WJ, Parrish RK. Trabeculectomy function after cataract extraction. Ophthalmology 1998; 105: 1928–35.

Cordeiro MF, Constable PH, Alexander RA, Bhattacharya SS, Khaw PT. Effect of varying the mitomycin-C treatment area in glaucoma filtration surgery in the rabbit. Invest Ophthalmol Vis Sci 1997; 38: 1639–46.

Costa VP, Smith M, Spaeth GL, Gandham S, Markovitz B. Loss of visual acuity after trabeculectomy. Ophthalmology 1993; 100: 599–612.

Crowston JG, Akbar AN, Constable PH et al. Antimetabolite-induced apoptosis in Tenon's capsule fibroblasts. Invest Ophthalmol Vis Sci 1998; 39: 449–54.

Doyle JW, Sherwood MB, Khaw PT, McGorray S, Smith MF. Intraoperative 5-fluorouracil for filtration surgery in the rabbit. Invest Ophthalmol Vis Sci 1993; 34: 3313–19.

Fannin LA, Schiffman JC, Budenz DL. Risk factors for hypotony maculopathy. Ophthalmology 2003; 110: 1185–91.

Fluorouracil Filtering Surgery Study Group. Five-year follow-up of the fluorouracil filtering surgery study group. Am J Ophthalmol 1996; 121: 349–66.

Gandolfi SA, Vecchi M, Braccio L. Decrease of intraocular pressure after subconjunctival injection of mitomycin in human glaucoma. Arch Ophthalmol 1995; 113: 582–5.

Greenfield DS, Suñer IJ, Miller MP et al. Endophthalmitis after filtering surgery with mitomycin. Arch Ophthalmol 1996; 114: 943–9.

Higginbotham EJ, Stevens RK, Musch DC et al. Bleb-related endophthalmitis after trabeculectomy with mitomycin C. Ophthalmology 1996; 103: 650–6.

Jampel HD, Quigley HA, Kerrigan-Baumrind LA et al. Risk factors for late-onset infection following glaucoma filtration surgery. Arch Ophthalmol 2001; 119: 1001–8.

Katz GJ, Higginbotham EJ, Lichter PR et al. Mitomycin C versus 5-fluorouracil in high-risk glaucoma filtering surgery. Extended follow-up. Ophthalmology 1995; 102: 1263–9.

Khaw PT, Doyle JW, Sherwood MB et al. Prolonged localised tissue effects from 5-minute exposures to fluorouracil and mitomycin C. Arch Ophthalmol 1993; 111: 263–7.

Khaw PT, Doyle JW, Sherwood MB, Smith MF, McGorray S. Effects of intraoperative 5-fluorouracil or mitomycin C on glaucoma filtering surgery in the rabbit. Ophthalmology 1993; 100: 367–72.

Lichter PR, Musch DC, Gillespie BW et al. Interim clinical outcomes in the Collaborative Initial Glaucoma Treatment Study comparing initial treatment randomized to medications or surgery. Ophthalmology 2001; 108: 1943–53.

Lochhead J, Casson RJ, Salmon JF. Long term effect on intraocular pressure of phacotrabeculectomy compared to trabeculectomy. Br J Ophthalmol 2003; 87: 850–2.

Palmer SS. Mitomycin as adjunct chemotherapy with trabeculectomy. Ophthalmology 1991; 98: 317–21.

Park H-J, Weitzman M, Caprioli J. Temporal corneal phacoemulsification combined with superior trabeculectomy. Arch Ophthalmol 1997; 115: 318–23.

Parrish RK, Schiffman JC, Feuer WJ, Heuer DK, The Fluorouracil Filtering Surgery Study Group. Prognosis and risk factors for early postoperative wound leaks after trabeculectomy with and without 5-fluorouracil. Am J Ophthalmol 2001; 132: 633–40.

Schraermeyer U, Diestelhorst M, Bieker A et al. Morphologic proof of the toxicity of mitomycin C on the ciliary body in relation to different application methods. Graefes Arch Clin Exp Ophthalmol 1999; 237: 593–600.

Schumer RA, Odrich SA. A scleral tunnel incision for trabeculectomy. Am J Ophthalmol 1995; 120: 528–30.

Singh K, Mehta K, Shaikh NM et al. Trabeculectomy with intraoperative mitomycin C versus 5-fluorouracil: prospective randomized clinical trial [In Process Citation]. Ophthalmology 2000; 107: 2305–9.

Wells AP, Cordeiro MF, Bunce C, Khaw PT. Cystic bleb formation and related complications in limbus versus fornix-based conjunctival flaps in paediatric and young adult trabeculectomy with mitomycin-C. Ophthalmology (in press).

Whittaker KW, Gillow JT, Cunliffe IA. Is the role of trabeculectomy in glaucoma management changing? Eye 2001; 15: 449–52.

Wilkins MR, Occleston NL, Kotecha A, Waters L, Khaw PT. Sponge delivery variables and tissue levels of 5-fluorouracil. Br J Ophthalmol 2000; 84: 92–7.

Zacharia PT, Deppermann SR, Schuman JS. Ocular hypotony after trabeculectomy with mitomycin C. Am J Ophthalmol 1993; 116: 314–26.

4. Aqueous drainage implants

Richard A Hill and George Baerveldt

INTRODUCTION

The implantation of an aqueous drainage device is usually an intermediary step between trabeculectomies with antimetabolites and cyclodestructive procedures, although in some situations it has been used as the first glaucoma surgery. Drainage device surgery is a type of filtering surgery where aqueous passively diffuses to a capsule over an implant. These implants are utilized in situations where a trabeculectomy is expected to have little chance for success. These situations include inflammatory and neovascular glaucoma, localized (post-operative) and generalized staphylomas (buphthalmic eyes), and a prior failed trabeculectomy with antimetabolites.

Although there are numerous devices, this chapter will focus on two devices that illustrate the major difference between aqueous drainage implants, whether they are flow-restricted (valved) or not. The Ahmed Glaucoma Valve™ (AGV) is representative of valved aqueous drainage implants, and the Baerveldt™ implant is representative of the non-valved class of aqueous drainage implants. Box 4.1 gives a list of the instruments required.

AHMED GLAUCOMA VALVES

The AGV is composed of a silicone drainage tube and a polypropylene or silicone reservoir body that houses a silicone elastomer valve membrane. The S-2 model and Ahmed Flexible plate (Figure 4.1) have a single plate (13 × 16 mm) with a surface area of 184 mm^2; the double plate version, the B-1, has a combined surface area of 364 mm^2 (a 12.2 × 14.8 mm non-valved plate and a 13 × 16 mm valved plate (Figure 4.2)). A pars plana adapter is also available (Figure 4.3). Drainage tubes for all the implants have a 0.64 mm external diameter with a 0.30 mm internal diameter. The valve-like mechanism is designed to open only if the intraocular pressure (IOP) exceeds 8 mmHg, and will, thus, prevent hypotony in the majority of cases.

Box 4.1 Instrumentation and supplies

Lieberman style wire lid speculum
Fine titanium needle driver
Pierse–Hoskins forceps
0.12 Castroviejo style forceps
Sub-miniature Wescott scissors
Full size Wescott scissors
Bonnacolto forceps
22/23-gauge needles
Long, angled McPherson tying forceps
Muscle hooks × 2
Pierse tip with tying platform forceps
6-0 polyglactin on S-29 needle
7-0 polypropylene on CV-1 or 8-0 nylon on TG-100-8 needle
8-0 polyglactin on TG-140-8
15° razor knife
Aqueous drainage implant or Glaucoma Drainage Device (GDD)
Biograft
Surgical sponges and cotton tip applicators
2 Mosquito-type hemostats
Bipolar cautery
27-gauge irrigating cannula with 3 ml syringe
Balanced salt solution (BSS)

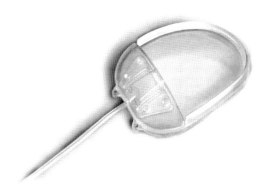

Figure 4.1 The Ahmed Glaucoma Valve model S-2 single plate (13 × 16 mm) with a surface area of 184 mm^2.

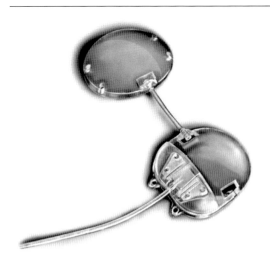

Figure 4.2 The Ahmed Glaucoma Valve model B-1. The combined surface area of the two plates is 364 mm² (12.2 × 14.8 mm non-valved plate; 13 × 16 mm valved plate).

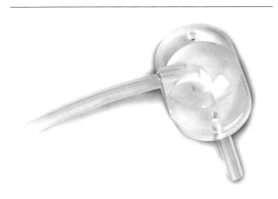

Figure 4.3 The Ahmed Glaucoma Valve pars plana adapter.

BAERVELDT IMPLANTS

Baerveldt implants are composed of barium sulfate impregnated, tumble-polished, 0.9-mm thick silicone plates. The plates are available in three sizes: a 250 (15 × 22 mm, 260 mm ± 5 mm (Figure 4.4)); a 350 (14 × 32 mm, 343 mm ± 7 mm; (Figure 4.4)) and a pars plana version based on the 350 model (Figure 4.5). The pars plana version has the

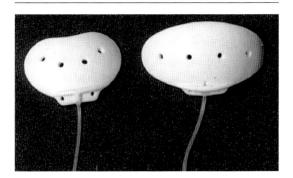

Figure 4.4 The Baerveldt glaucoma implant model 250 (a). The plate measures 15 × 22 mm with a surface area of 260 mm ± 5 mm. The Baerveldt glaucoma implant model 350 (b). The plate measures 14 × 32 mm with a surface area of 343 mm ± 7 mm.

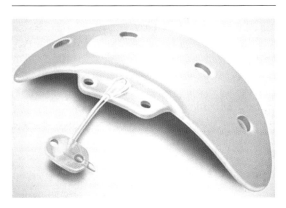

Figure 4.5 The Baerveldt glaucoma implant pars plana version. The plate (model 350) measures 14 × 32 mm with a surface area of 343 mm ± 7 mm.

Hoffman elbow, which of consists of a small episcleral plate with two suture holes and a 5.1-mm semirigid, tapered and beveled cannula, that is inserted through a pars plana sclerotomy. This cannula is angled posteriorly at 105° to prevent lenticular contact. The drainage tube has the same dimensions as the AGV. The anterior flange has two large suture holes. The tube crosses the small flange area and passes through the ridge. The straight 10-mm long ridge was designed to be used in patients with encircling elements from previous retinal surgery. There are also fenestrations in the plate which allow tissue growth between the capsule walls in order to limit the elevation of the surrounding capsule.

SURGICAL ACCESS: GENERAL CONSIDERATIONS

In order of preference, drainage devices are placed in the superior/temporal, superior/nasal and inferior/temporal quadrants. Placement in the superior nasal quadrant is associated with an increased incidence of a pseudo Brown's syndrome (see the section on complications). When aqueous drainage implants are placed in the superior/nasal quadrant, it should be kept in mind that the optic nerve is closer to the limbus in this quadrant than the superior/temporal and inferior/temporal quadrants.

In a large number of patients retrobulbar anesthesia will yield poor analgesia and akinesia. The anesthesia can be supplemented with topical tetracaine prior to placing the corneal traction suture; once the sub-Tenon's tunnel is dissected, an additional 1–2 ml of local anesthetic can be instilled into this area with a blunt cannula.

The corneal traction suture (Figure 4.6) consists of 6-0 polyglactin on an S-29 strabismus needle. It is passed through the peripheral cornea at approximately 50% depth. In the event of anterior chamber perforation the polyglactin suture should be withdrawn. The puncture wound is usually small enough and beveled enough to seal spontaneously. A second track can be made slightly above the first track. The polyglactin suture is then twisted and clipped inferiorly to the drapes with a small mosquito clamp. A corneal light protector should always be used to protect the patient's macula (Figure 4.7). In many advanced glaucoma cases the macula represents the majority of the functioning retina. The choice between a fornix-based or limbus-based peritomy is primarily the preference of the operating surgeon. However, there are a few practical points to consider. The first point is relative to how much limbal scarring is present. In cases with extensive limbal scarring, a fornix-based peritomy with long radial relaxing incisions 120° apart is preferred and gives good exposure to the surgical site. Radial relaxing incisions are made long enough to give access to the recti muscles. A radial relaxing incision is made by picking the tissue up with nontoothed forceps in a radial fashion and pressing the open tips of blunt Wescott scissors down to the surface of the globe and closing them (Figure 4.8).

A short limbus-based peritomy with the incision 3–4 mm posterior to the limbus may also be used.

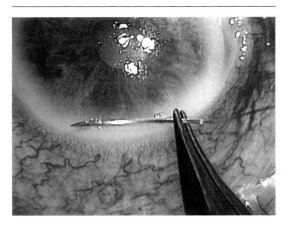

Figure 4.6 The corneal traction suture consists of a 6-0 polyglactin on an S-29 strabismus needle. It is passed through the peripheral cornea at approximately 80% depth.

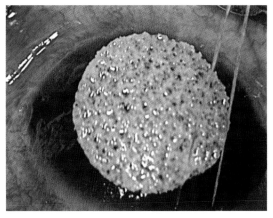

Figure 4.7 A corneal light protector should always be used to protect the patient's macula.

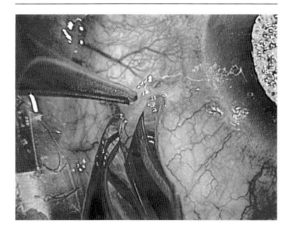

Figure 4.8 A radial relaxing incision is made by picking the conjunctiva and Tenon's up with nontoothed forceps in a radial fashion.

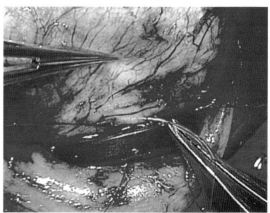

Figure 4.9 Sutures used to secure drainage implants should be nonabsorbable such as Prolene on a tapered vascular type needle (7-0 or 8-0 polypropylene on a CV-1). Alternatively, an 8-0 nylon suture on a spatula needle such as a TG100-8 can also be used (shown).

The advantage of this mini-limbus based peritomy is that it gives good access to the area where the drainage device will be placed and minimizes the cumbersome nature of the longer flaps associated with fornix-based conjunctival flaps. When dissecting between rectus muscles, great care should be taken not to enter orbital fat. This can result in orbital fat syndrome with strabismus.

SECURING THE DRAINAGE EXOPLANT

GENERAL CONSIDERATIONS

It is important to minimize the amount of implanted hardware in the superior nasal quadrant as this is known to induce a pseudo Brown's syndrome. When implants are placed in the superonasal quadrant, it is important to not engage or injure the superior oblique tendon. This is an important consideration for all implants. Sutures used to secure implants should be nonabsorbable, such as Prolene, on a tapered vascular type needle (7-0 or 8-0 polypropylene on a CV-1). The tapered needle has the practical advantage of decreasing the risk of ocular perforation. Alternatively an 8-0 nylon suture on a spatula needle such as a TG100-8

can also be used (Figure 4.9). If this needle is used, care must be taken not to allow the side-cutting needle to rotate off its parallel arc to the sclera because of the risk of scleral perforation. If the sclera is staphylomatous or there is a history of scleritis, the sutures can be passed through the recti muscle tendons at their insertions.

AGV

The AGV should not be held with forceps over the valve cover body (Figure 4.10) as this may damage the retaining rivets on the valve cover, allowing fibrovascular ingrowth with subsequent device failure. The AGV is also longer in an anterior/posterior direction than the Baerveldt implant, and it should not be implanted too far posteriorly as the optic nerve can be compromised. Generally it is implanted 8–10 mm posterior to the limbus and the temporal quadrant is preferred. If either device is implanted nasally, there is a higher incidence of strabismus and a shorter path to the optic nerve. The AGV should be implanted no further than 8 mm from the limbus when placed nasally because of the risk of compromising the optic nerve.

In the case of the double-plate AGV, a longer (10:00–2:00) fornix-based peritomy or a limbal/

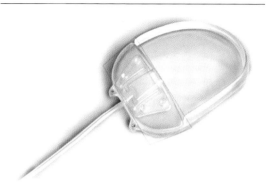

Figure 4.10 The Ahmed valve should not be held with forceps over the valve cover body as this may damage the retaining rivets of the valve cover. This allows fibrovascular ingrowth with subsequent device failure.

fornix-based combination may be used. A Tenon's traction suture will ensure good exposure (Figure 4.11). The connecting tube may be passed either under the superior rectus muscle or over the superior rectus muscle, but it is very important that no intervening Tenon's tissue be present. In earlier models, this tissue could easily disconnect the two plates. A modified version of the double plated is less easily disconnected. This modified version of the connecting clip may be sprung open for easy insertion of the connecting tube by sliding one tine of a small forceps into this clip (Figure 4.12).

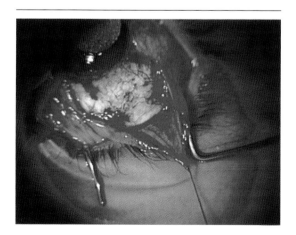

Figure 4.11 A Tenon's traction suture will help ensure excellent exposure. Pass the needle of the second half of the corneal traction suture through the posterior edge of Tenon's capsule.

BAERVELDT IMPLANT

When placing the Baerveldt implant, the surgeon needs to isolate the lateral and superior rectus muscles with muscle hooks. Either the superior or lateral rectus is engaged with one muscle hook and a second muscle hook is placed under the belly of the same muscle. The implant is held lengthwise by large nontoothed forceps such as Bonnacolto forceps (Figure 4.13) and placed deeply (about 70% of its length) behind the lateral or superior rectus. The

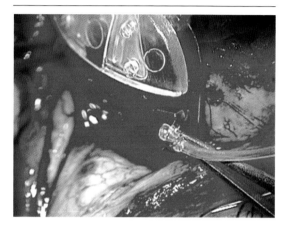

Figure 4.12 A retaining clip is used to attach the drainage tube of the second plate. This clip may be sprung open for easy insertion of the connecting tube by sliding one tine of a small forceps into this clip.

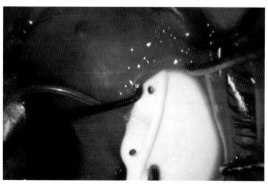

Figure 4.13 To place the Baerveldt implant, it is held lengthwise with large nontoothed forceps such as Bonnacolto forceps (Figure 4.15) and set deeply (about 70% of its length) behind the lateral or superior rectus.

muscle hook is then used to elevate the muscle so the implant can then be tucked behind the muscle and centered between the recti muscles (Figure 4.14). The implant is then sutured to the scleral surface at a distance of 10–12 mm posterior to the limbus.

DRAINAGE TUBE PLACEMENT

GENERAL CONSIDERATIONS

For both devices, the drainage tube is trimmed to the correct length to allow the tube to penetrate into the anterior chamber approximately 1–2 mm (Figure 4.15). The exception to this is neovascular glaucoma where florid rubeosis is present, and a high chance for a fibrovascular cicatrix is present. In this case, the tube tip can extend into the pupillary space, or the tube can be placed through the pars plana if the eye has had a vitrectomy.

The tubes are trimmed with a bevel facing the corneal endothelium to minimize the chance of iris incarceration. With either aqueous drainage device, the presence of a global or local staphyloma may necessitate the use of a smaller fistulizing needle (for example a 25-gauge needle for the AGV and a 23-gauge needle for the Baerveldt) to prevent excessive aqueous run-off around the tube and hypotony

(Figures 4.16, 4.17). When the fistulous tract is created, it is important that the eye does not rotate as the needle track is made. The tract should be parallel to and just anterior to the iris. When using a 22-gauge needle, the tract should be made expeditiously as the angled lumen of the needle is longer than the corneal thickness and the anterior chamber will decompress. There is a high risk of corneal

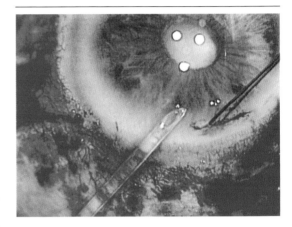

Figure 4.15 For both devices, the drainage tube is then trimmed to the correct length to allow the tube to penetrate into the anterior chamber approximately 1–2 mm.

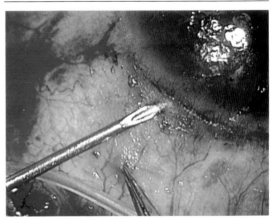

Figure 4.16 With either aqueous drainage device, the presence of a global or local staphyloma may necessitate the use of a smaller fistulizing needle (25-gauge Ahmed; 23-gauge Baerveldt) to prevent excessive peri-tube aqueous run-off and hypotony. When the fistulous tract is created it is important that the eye does not rotate as the needle track is made.

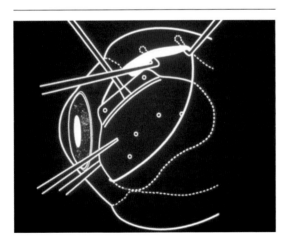

Figure 4.14 The muscle hook is used to elevate the muscle so the implant can then be tucked behind the muscle and centered between the recti muscles.

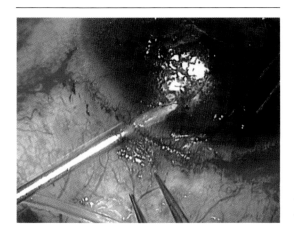

Figure 4.17 The track should be made expeditiously as the angled lumen of the needle is longer than the corneal thickness and the anterior chamber will decompress.

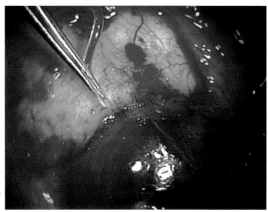

Figure 4.18 The drainage tube may be passed through the fistulous tract either with one of a number of special forceps or simply with the use of long, angled tying forceps. These should compress a length of tubing equal to their jaw length with approximately a millimeter extending beyond the tips of the instrument.

transplant failure after placement of aqueous drainage implants and care should be taken when placing the tube. The drainage tube may be passed through the fistulous tract cither with one of a number of special forceps or simply with the use of long, angled tying forceps. These should compress a length of tubing equal to their jaw length with about a millimeter extending beyond the tips of the forceps (Figure 4.18). After placement, the drainage tube is then secured to the episcleral surface with 8-0 caliber absorbable sutures (Figure 4.19).

AGV

The AGV will not function unless it is primed by cannulating (27-gauge cannula) the drainage tube and irrigating a small amount of BSS through the valve mechanism (Figure 4.20). This is an extremely important step. The tube is placed in the anterior chamber through a 23-gauge needle track starting about 1 mm posterior to the limbus. If a second needle track is made, the first track should be closed with a 10-0 nylon suture.

THE BAERVELDT IMPLANT

In the case of a nonvalved device, maneuvers must be utilized to minimize chances of post-

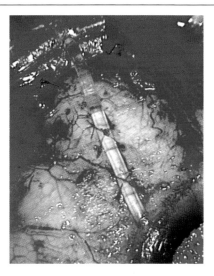

Figure 4.19 After placement of the drainage tube in the anterior chamber, it is secured to the episcleral surface with 8-0 caliber absorbable sutures.

operative hyper- or hypotension in the immediate postoperative period. The drainage tube may be ligated with an absorbable suture, just in front of its origin from the aqueous drainage device. The time period before suture lysis varies with suture size: 7-0

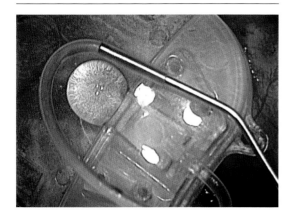

Figure 4.20 The Ahmed Glaucoma Valve will not function unless it is primed by cannulating (27-gauge cannula) the drainage tube and irrigating a small amount of BSS through the valve mechanism.

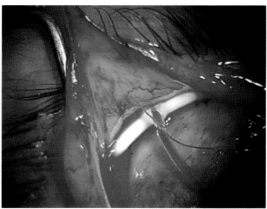

Figure 4.21 To prevent postoperative hypotony, the drainage tube of the Baerveldt implant must be ligated anterior to its origin from the implant plate. Either 7-0 polyglactin (4–6 weeks until rupture) or 8-0 polyglactin (2–4 weeks until rupture) may be used.

polyglactin, generally ruptures after 4–6 weeks and 8-0 polyglactin, after 2–4 weeks (Figure 4.21). The occlusion of the tube may be demonstrated by attempted irrigation of BSS through a 27-gauge cannula inserted into the tube. The ligated tube is then passed into the anterior chamber through a 22-gauge needle track, which starts about 1 mm posterior to the limbus. If tube malposition is noted, a step ladder technique of reintroducing the needle in ½ mm steps anteriorly or posteriorly to the original opening may be done. This will allow the surgeon to obtain proper needle/tube position without injury to the contents of the anterior chamber.

The larger bore needle tract may be selected with the Baerveldt implant to allow some leakage of aqueous around the silicone drainage tube. In addition, two relief slits anterior to the ligature may be made in the drainage tube with the needle on the 7-0/8-0 polyglactin suture. These are double perforating cut (Figure 4.22) that are best placed after the tube is secured to the scleral surface and help prevent postoperative elevation of IOP.

Alternatively, another technique known as a ripcord may be used (Figure 4.23). This involves the use of a 4-0 Prolene suture placed either into the drainage tube in a retrograde fashion or laid parallel to the drainage tube. The drainage tube lumen is then ligated with a 7-0 polyglactin suture. The needle of the Prolene suture is then passed subcon-

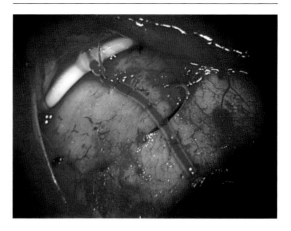

Figure 4.22 After the Baerveldt drainage tube is ligated, two double perforating relief slits are cut in the drainage tube to minimize chances for postoperative hypertension. The perforations may be made with the needle on the 7-0/8-0 polyglactin suture material.

junctivally and inferiorly so that the suture exits the conjunctiva about 4 mm posteriorly to the limbus in the inferior fornix; it is cut flush to the conjunctiva. The suture is removed after the implant undergoes encapsulation, because then the capsule will offer resistance to the outflow of aqueous from the eye.

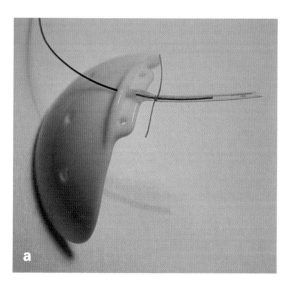 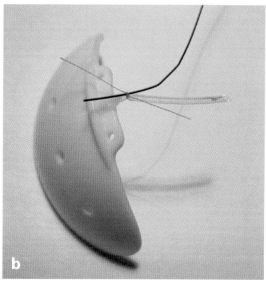

Figure 4.23 (a,b) A ripcord may also be used. This involves the use of a 4-0 prolene suture placed either into the drainage tube in a retrograde fashion or laid parallel to the drainage tube. The drainage tube lumen is then compressed with a 7-0 polyglactin suture to form an occlusion. The needle of the Prolene suture is then passed subconjunctivally and inferiorly so that the suture exits the conjunctiva about 4 mm posteriorly to the limbus in the inferior fornix and cut flush. The suture is removed after the implant undergoes encapsulation, which offers resistance to outflow of aqueous.

PARS PLANA PLACEMENT OF THE DRAINAGE TUBE

There are certain clinical situations where it may be desirable to place the drainage tube through the pars plana. These situations include the presence of a shallow anterior chamber, aphakia, penetrating keratoplasty, and/or an extensive anterior staphyloma/scar. Pars plana insertion does require an adequate vitrectomy with trimming of the vitreous skirt back to its insertion. The Baerveldt implant with the Hoffman elbow is easier to use than the implant without the elbow when attempting pars plana insertion. Even when gas is placed into the eye, investigators have found that the frequency of postoperative hypotony is less when the tube is ligated. Thus, it is recommended to ligate the tube with an absorbable suture.

SECURING THE BIOGRAFT: GENERAL CONSIDERATIONS

A freehand biograft is fashioned to cover any staphylomas resulting from any previous trabeculectomy or cataract surgery as well as to cover the drainage tube to help prevent its extrusion through the conjunctiva. A notch may be cut in the posterior edge of the biograft so as to allow lysis of any ligating polyglactin suture with an Argon laser as needed. The biograft may be created from any of a number of materials, the most popular of which are donor sclera or pericardium (Figure 4.24).

CLOSING THE PERITOMY: GENERAL CONSIDERATIONS

Care must be taken with wound approximation to prevent epithelial ingrowth as well as poor wound closure especially with fornix-based peritomies. Typically, residual conjunctiva at the limbus should

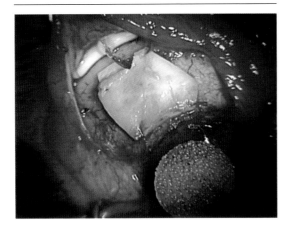

Figure 4.24 A biograft is placed to reinforce a thinned limbus and to prevent extrusion of the drainage tube. The biograft may be any of a number of materials, the most popular of which are donor sclera and donor pericardium. A posterior notch in the sclera graft will facilitate laser sututelysis, if desired.

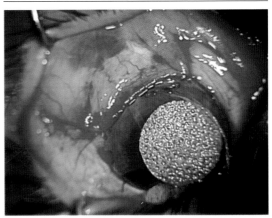

Figure 4.25 Closure of the peritomy with scleral anchoring sutures. When the tension is correct there will be a groove in the tissue about 2 mm behind the leading edge.

BAERVELDT IMPLANT

The main issue regarding the postoperative care of nonvalved implants is the release of the ligature. In cases where a ripcord was used, this can usually be removed in 7–10 days because of very elevated eye pressures although its removal in 3–6 weeks is usually safer and limits the exposure of the eye to transient hypotony and its sequelae. The 8-0 polyglactin ligature normally releases between 2–4 weeks and the 7-0 polyglactin ligature releases around 4–6 weeks. The suture can be lysed either in the operating room or with a laser if the ligature is visible at the posterior margin of the biograft and the eye pressures are very elevated.

be trimmed and removed carefully. The fornix-based flap can be reapproximated with interrupted polyglactin sutures which engage the sclera in one of the needle bites. In this way the conjunctiva can be firmly anchored and good wound healing is assured (Figure 4.25). In the case of a device such as a Baerveldt implant it is very important to close the conjunctiva in a watertight fashion as this will allow additional resistance to outflow if leakage around the drainage tube or if leakage through the drainage release slits is excessive.

POSTOPERATIVE CARE

GENERAL CONSIDERATIONS

At the conclusion of the surgery, antibiotics and steroids are administered subconjunctivally and the eye is patched. The following day, the patient is started on topical antibiotics and steroids. In cases of severe inflammation, topical steroids may be used hourly; otherwise they may be used every 2 hours and tapered as the conjunctival injection decreases. An elevated IOP can be lowered, if necessary, by restarting preoperative glaucoma medications.

TREATMENT OF COMPLICATIONS

INADVERTENT OCULAR PERFORATION

Needle passes for securing the plates or exoplants are posterior to the ora serrata. If the surgeon inadvertently rotates a spatula-type needle into the eye during the scleral pass or makes a pass too deep through this thin area of sclera, an ocular perforation with retinal hole formation can occur. Should this occur, a cryo spot with a cryoprobe should be placed over the site. The exoplant may then be tightly sutured to sclera in a slightly anterior position producing a buckling effect.

EXTRUDING IMPLANTED MATERIAL

At first one may notice that the tissue over the exoplant or tube has thinned. When the vasculature in the overlying tissue disappears, this is an indication for the surgeon to revise this area with a new biograft or to reposition the plate because extrusion is imminent. Preemptive surgery is indicated to minimize the chances of endophthalmitis. Obvious causes for extrusion should be sought such as a plate placed too anteriorly where there is constant interaction with the eyelid. Often there may be no obvious reason. One option for repairing extrusions is to use the Persian carpet maneuver. In this technique the surgeon undermines and mobilizes the tissue surrounding the defect over the plate or tube. A biograft is rolled up like a carpet and passed through the defect and unfurled under this area. The defect is then closed, incorporating the biograft for additional strength. The authors' preferred material in this situation is donor sclera. The authors strongly urge that only resorbable sutures be used to close conjunctiva and secure the biograft. Recurrent exoplant extrusion should alert the surgeon to the possibility of epithelial ingrowth.

STRABISMUS

The strabismus produced by aqueous drainage implants is usually secondary to a mass effect. A less frequent cause is entering into the orbital fat and causing fat fibrosis syndrome. Care must also be taken not to injure the rectus muscles during the retrobulbar injection or during surgery and not to entrap the tendon of the superior oblique. The mass effect can produce an incomitant strabismus by limiting movement of the eye in the direction of the implant. Typically a hypotropia with an exotropia is produced by a superior/temporal implant while pseudo Brown's syndrome may be produced by a superior/nasal implant. The incidence of strabismus with the Baerveldt implant has deceased with the incorporation of fenestrations or holes in the implant plate. These fenestrations allow ingrowth of fibrous tissue which decrease the volume and height of the filtering capsule bleb. Strabismus following valve implantation is difficult to treat. If prisms and strabismus surgery fail, another effective option for treatment of the motility disorder is removal of the drainage device, but this is not often a sight-preserving option in this group of patients.

TUBE-RELATED COMPLICATIONS

Tube malposition is best prevented at the time of tube placement by proper orientation of the needle track into the anterior chamber. Tubes that are too close to the iris or lens can produce inflammation, hemorrhage or cataract, while those that are too close to the cornea, may decrease endothelial cell counts – which may lead to graft failure in eyes with a penetrating keratoplasty. If tube malposition occurs during surgery, the tube should be withdrawn and the needle track closed with a 10-0 nylon suture to avoid hypotony. An additional tract can then be made. If the drainage tube is cut intraoperatively, it can be repaired with the Teflon sheath of an angiocath or more preferably with available repair kits (New World Medical, Rancho Cucamungo, CA). Postoperatively, if the tube retracts or extends further into the eye, the tube may be revised by either shortening or using an extending repair kit (Figure 4.26).

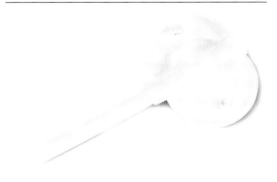

Figure 4.26 If a drainage tube is cut too short or retracts postoperatively the tube may be revised by using a drainage tube extending repair kit.

CONCLUSION

Drainage devices have an important role in the management of patients with glaucoma. Although they are becoming more popular, there are still numerous complications, which the surgeon can avoid with appropriate intraoperative techniques and postoperative follow-up.

FURTHER READING

Ayyala RS, Zurakowski D, Smith JA et al. A clinical study of the Ahmed Glaucoma Valve Implant in advanced glaucoma. Ophthalmology 1998; 105: 1968–76.

Britt MT, LaBree LD, Lloyd MA et al. Randomized clinical trial of the 350-mm^2 versus the 500-mm^2 Baerveldt implant: longer term results: is bigger better? Ophthalmology 1999; 106: 2312–18.

Budenz DL, Sakamoto D, Eliezer R, Varma R, Heuer DK. Two-staged Baerveldt glaucoma implant for childhood glaucoma associated with Sturge–Weber syndrome. Ophthalmology 2000; 107: 2105–10.

Coleman AL, Hill R, Wilson MR et al. Initial clinical experience with the Ahmed Glaucoma Valve implant. Am J Ophthalmol 1995; 120: 23–31.

Da Mata A, Burk SE, Netland PA et al. Management of uveitic glaucoma with Ahmed glaucoma valve implantation. Ophthalmology 1999; 106: 2168–72.

Desatnik HR, Foster RE, Rockwood EJ et al. Management of glaucoma implants occluded by vitreous incarceration. J Glaucoma 2000; 9: 311–16.

Djodeyre MR, Peralta Calvo J, Abelairas Gomez J. Clinical evaluation and risk factors of time to failure of Ahmed Glaucoma Valve implant in pediatric patients. Ophthalmology 2001; 108: 614–20.

Englert JA, Freedman SF, Cox TA. The Ahmed valve in refractory pediatric glaucoma. Am J Ophthalmol 1999; 127: 34–42.

Gedde SJ, Scott IU, Tabandeh H et al. Late endophthalmitis associated with glaucoma drainage implants. Ophthalmology 2001; 108: 1323–7.

Hamush NG, Coleman AL, Wilson MR. Ahmed glaucoma valve implant for management of glaucoma in Sturge–Weber syndrome. Am J Ophthalmol 1999; 128: 758–60.

Heuer DK, Lloyd MA, Abrams DA et al. Which is better? One or two? A randomized clinical trial of single-plate Molteno implantation for glaucomas in aphakia and pseudophakia. Ophthalmology 1992; 99: 1512–19.

Hill RA. Tenon's traction sutures: an aid for trabeculectomy and aqueous drainage device implantation. J Glaucoma 2002; 11: 529–30.

Hill R, Brown R, Heuer DK. Laser suture lysis for non-valved aqueous drainage implants. J Glaucoma 2003; 12: 390–1.

Hill RA, Heuer DK, Baerveldt G, Minckler DS, Martone JF. Molteno implantation for glaucoma in young patients. Ophthalmology 1991; 98: 1042–6.

Hill RA, Pirouzian A, Liaw L. Pathophysiology of and prophylaxis against late Ahmed Glaucoma Valve occlusion. Am J Ophthalmol 2000; 129: 608–12.

Huang MC, Netland PA, Coleman AL et al. Intermediate-term clinical experience with the Ahmed Glaucoma Valve implant. Am J Ophthalmol 1999; 127: 27–33.

Hodkin MJ, Goldblatt WS, Burgoyne CF, Ball SF, Insler MS. Early clinical experience with the Baerveldt implant in complicated glaucomas. Am J Ophthalmol 1995; 120: 32–40.

Kwon YH, Taylor JM, Hong S et al. Long-term results of eyes with penetrating keratoplasty and glaucoma drainage tube implant. Ophthalmology 2001; 108: 272–8.

Law SK, Kalenak JW, Connor TB Jr et al. Retinal complications after aqueous shunt surgical procedures for glaucoma. Arch Ophthalmol 1996; 114: 1473–80.

Leen MM, Witkop GS, George DP. Anatomic considerations in the implantation of the Ahmed glaucoma valve. Arch Ophthalmol 1996; 114(2): 223–4.

Lloyd MA, Sedlak T, Heuer DK et al. Clinical experience with the single-plate Molteno implant in complicated glaucomas. Update of a pilot study. Ophthalmology 1992; 99: 679–87.

Lloyd MA, Baerveldt G, Fellenbaum PS et al. Intermediate-term results of a randomized clinical trial of the 350- versus the 500-mm^2 Baerveldt implant. Ophthalmology 1994; 101: 1456–63; discussion 1463–4.

Lloyd MA, Baerveldt G, Heuer DK, Minckler DS, Martone JF. Initial clinical experience with the Baerveldt implant in complicated glaucomas. Ophthalmology 1994; 101: 640–50.

Luttrell JK, Avery R, Baerveldt G, Easley K. Initial experience with pneumatically stented Baerveldt implant modified for pars plana insertion for complicated glaucoma. Ophthalmology 2000; 107: 143–50.

McDonnell PJ, Robin JB, Schanzlin DJ et al. Molteno implant for control of glaucoma in eyes after penetrating keratoplasty. Ophthalmology 1988; 95: 364–9.

Melamed S, Goldenfeld M, Barequet I. Anatomic considerations in the implantation of the Ahmed glaucoma valve. Arch Ophthalmol 1996; 114: 1298–9.

Minckler DS, Heuer DK, Hasty B et al. Clinical experience with the single-plate Molteno implant in complicated glaucomas. Ophthalmology 1988; 95: 1181–8.

Munoz M, Parrish RK 2nd. Strabismus following implantation of Baerveldt drainage devices. Arch Ophthalmol 1993; 111: 1096–9.

Netland PA, Walton DS. Glaucoma drainage implants in pediatric patients. Ophthalmic Surg 1993; 24: 723–9.

Nguyen QH, Budenz DL, Parrish RK 2nd. Complications of Baerveldt glaucoma drainage implants. Arch Ophthalmol 1998; 116: 571–5.

Scott IU, Gedde SJ, Budenz DL et al. Baerveldt drainage implants in eyes with a preexisting scleral buckle. Arch Ophthalmol 2000; 118: 1509–13.

Sidoti PA, Minckler DS, Baerveldt G, Lee PP, Heuer DK. Epithelial ingrowth and glaucoma drainage implants. Ophthalmology 1994; 101: 872–5.

Sidoti PA, Dunphy TR, Baerveldt G et al. Experience with the Baerveldt glaucoma implant in treating neovascular glaucoma. Ophthalmology 1995; 102: 1107–18.

Sidoti PA, Mosny AY, Ritterband DC, Seedor JA. Pars plana tube insertion of glaucoma drainage implants and penetrating keratoplasty in patients with coexisting glaucoma and corneal disease. Ophthalmology 2001; 108: 1050–8.

Siegner SW, Netland PA, Urban RC Jr et al. Clinical experience with the Baerveldt glaucoma drainage implant. Ophthalmology 1995; 102: 1298–307.

Smith SL, Starita RJ, Fellman RL, Lynn JR. Early clinical experience with the Baerveldt 350-mm^2 glaucoma implant and associated extraocular muscle imbalance. Ophthalmology 1993; 100: 914–18.

Smith MF, Doyle JW, Sherwood MB. Comparison of the Baerveldt glaucoma implant with the double-plate Molteno drainage implant. Arch Ophthalmol 1995; 113: 444–7.

Smith MF, Doyle JW, Fanous MM. Modified aqueous drainage implants in the treatment of complicated glaucomas in eyes with pre-existing episcleral bands. Ophthalmology 1998; 105: 2237–42.

Topouzis F, Coleman AL, Choplin N et al. Follow-up of the original cohort with the Ahmed glaucoma valve implant. Am J Ophthalmol 1999; 128: 198–204.

Trible JR, Brown DB. Occlusive ligature and standardized fenestration of a Baerveldt tube with and without antimetabolites for early postoperative intraocular pressure control. Ophthalmology 1998; 105: 2243–50.

Wilson MR, Mendis U, Smith SD, Paliwal A. Ahmed glaucoma valve implant vs. trabeculectomy in the surgical treatment of glaucoma: a randomized clinical trial. Am J Ophthalmol 2000; 130: 267–3.

5. Nonpenetrating glaucoma surgery

Tarek Shaarawy and André Mermoud

INTRODUCTION

The first suggestion of a disease associated with a rise in intraocular pressure (IOP) and thus corresponding to what is now known as glaucoma occurs in the Arabian writings of Shamsad-Deen of Cairo, thirteenth century Egyptian ophthalmologist; he described a 'headache of the pupil, an illness associated with pain in the eye, hemicrania and dullness of the humours, and followed by dilatation of the pupil and cataract; if it becomes chronic, tenseness of the eye and blindness supervened'. Ever since then, the mainstay of glaucoma therapy has been to lower IOP, medically or surgically.

Trabeculectomy has been the gold standard of glaucoma surgery ever since Dr Sugar in 1961 and Dr Cairns in 1968 suggested a shift from the then widely practiced full-thickness glaucoma filtering procedures. The use of a superficial flap was of paramount importance in creating resistance to aqueous outflow, lowering the incidence of postoperative hypotony as well as offering protection against the catastrophic occurrence of endophthalmitis. Through the years the evidence has mounted showing that trabeculectomy is perhaps not the 'holy grail' in the quest for an ideal surgery for glaucoma. Most surgeons prefer to delay surgery because of the potential vision-threatening complications of classical trabeculectomy, with or without antimetabolites. Complications include hypotony, hyphema, flat anterior chamber, choroidal effusion or hemorrhage, surgery-induced cataract, and bleb failure. In spite of the tendency to delay surgery, it remains a very effective way of lowering IOP. Some authors hypothesize that if the safety margin of glaucoma surgery could be increased significantly without sacrificing efficacy, surgical intervention for glaucoma might be considered earlier.

Mikhail Leonidovich Krasnov, of the former USSR, paved the ground for nonpenetrating filtering surgery, when he published his pioneer work on what he called sinusotomy. Several techniques have since evolved, probably the most popular of which are deep sclerectomy with collagen implant (DSCI) and viscocanalostomy.

PRINCIPLES OF NONPENETRATING FILTERING SURGERY

The main idea behind nonpenetrating filtering surgery is to somehow surgically enhance the natural aqueous outflow channels, rather than to create a new and possibly overly effective drainage site. Avoidance of penetration of the anterior chamber should allow the anterior segment to recover more quickly with less risk of hypotony and its sequelae.

In primary, and in most cases of secondary, open angle glaucoma, the main resistance to aqueous outflow is thought to be located at the level of the juxtacanalicular trabeculum and the inner wall of Schlemm's canal. These two anatomic structures can be removed. This technique was first proposed by Zimmermann, and he used the term ab externo trabeculectomy to describe it (Figure 5.1).

Another way to increase the aqueous outflow in a patient with restricted posterior trabeculum outflow is to remove the corneal stroma behind the anterior trabeculum and Descemet's membrane. This has been called deep sclerectomy and was first described by Fyodorov and Kozlov (Figure 5.2). After deep sclerectomy, the main outflow of aqueous occurs at the level of the anterior trabeculum and Descemet's membrane, the so-called trabeculo-Descemet's membrane (TDM) (see Figure 5.2).

In viscocanalostomy, described by Stegmann, the aqueous filters through the TDM into the scleral space, as in deep sclerectomy, but it does not form a subconjunctival filtering bleb because the superficial scleral flap is tightly closed. From the scleral space, the aqueous reaches the Schlemm's

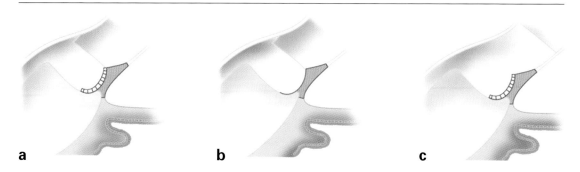

a **b** **c**

Figure 5.1 Comparison of sinusotomy, deep sclerectomy, and ab externo trabulectomy in pig eyes. (a) Sinusotomy. A lamellar band of the sclera is removed and Schlemm's canal is opened over 120° from 10 to 12 o'clock. The inner wall of Schlemm's canal is not touched. (b) Ab externo trabulectomy. (c) Deep sclerectomy. Arrows indicate aqueous dynamics.

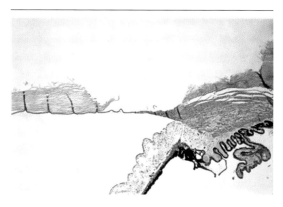

Figure 5.2 Histology of the trabuleco-Descemet's membrane dyed with ferritin. The dye is present in the anterior part of the trabecular meshwork (human eye).

canal ostia, which are surgically opened and dilated with a viscoelastic substance.

INDICATIONS FOR NONPENETRATING GLAUCOMA SURGERY

In general, the indications for nonpenetrating glaucoma surgery (NPGS) are wider and more inclusive than those for classical trabeculectomies. The reasons for this statement are twofold: first, NPGS is safer but not less efficient (when performed by a NPGS-trained surgeon) than trabeculectomies;

secondly, NPGS is indicated in certain types of glaucoma where trabeculectomies normally fail or are not possible.

Until the advent of NPGS, penetrating glaucoma surgery was generally considered the last resort in the treatment of glaucoma. When medical and laser therapies failed to lower IOP to an acceptable level, glaucoma specialists resorted to surgery to halt the progression of the disease. NPGS with its lower complication rate can be offered earlier in the course of the disease. In fact, NPGS can be offered as a first-line treatment in cases where it is obvious that medical treatment will be insufficient for lowering the IOP to acceptable levels. This is particularly important in the younger glaucoma patient who has a longer lifespan and cannot be medically treated for several decades. Furthermore, glaucoma surgery in general, and NPGS in particular, is more successful in glaucoma patients who were not exposed to medical treatment. The noxious effects of topical medications on the conjunctiva are well documented. The conjunctival tissues undergo a scarring process when exposed to certain topical medications. Scarred conjunctiva, as found in patients who have been medically treated for years, is less amenable to the formation of a healthy diffuse bleb than 'virgin' conjunctiva. It is possible that even the trabeculum undergoes biochemical–structural changes after years of medical treatment, rendering it less responsive to NPGS. It is, therefore, logical to propose NPGS earlier than later when the chances of favorable outcomes are greater. The previous teaching of 'first medical and laser treatment and then surgical treatment' has to be reviewed in the light of the promising outcomes of NPGS.

OPEN ANGLE GLAUCOMA

Open angle glaucoma (OAG) is the commonest type of glaucoma and presents the best indication for NPGS. Furthermore, NPGS targets the presumed site of pathology, namely the trabecular meshwork. During NPGS, the trabeculum is exposed and examined by the surgeon who can evaluate the amount of filtration in vivo. The experienced surgeon can compare the appearance of the trabeculum and its filtration capacity with cases he or she has done in the past. The site of the resistance to aqueous outflow is presumed to be the juxtacanalicular trabeculum and the inner wall of Schlemm's canal. During NPGS, the surgeon attempts to improve filtration by 'reconditioning' the trabecular meshwork. Scraping, thinning out, and peeling the posterior trabeculum improve filtration. NPGS has the advantage of possibly being less cataractogenic than trabeculectomy.

GLAUCOMA PATIENTS WITH HIGH MYOPIA

Conventional glaucoma surgery in patients with high myopia carries an especially high risk of complications because of the abnormal dimensions of the globe. Choroidal detachments and consequent shallow anterior chambers, occur in 10–15% of trabeculectomies performed in highly myopic glaucoma patients.

Hamel and coworkers in 2001 studied NPGS in highly myopic glaucoma patients. Thirty-eight percent had IOP below 21 mmHg without medication 48 months after surgery. Eighty-one percent of the patients achieved an IOP below 21 mmHg with or without medications (qualified success rate) 48 months after surgery. In this series, only two patients developed choroidal detachments, one of which was secondary to blunt trauma to the operated eye six days after surgery. This incidence is lower than the 10–15% rate reported for classical trabeculectomy. NPGS appears to have safer outcome in glaucoma patients with high myopia because of the gradual intraoperative IOP reduction.

PIGMENTARY GLAUCOMA

Three main reasons make NPGS an attractive treatment for pigmentary glaucoma (Figure 5.3): (i) the high resistance of this condition to medical treatment, (ii) the fact that NPGS targets the site of pathology, namely the pigment-loaded trabecular meshwork, and (iii) the fact that pigmentary glaucoma occurs more frequently in young, myopic male adults to whom it is more desirable to offer a safe surgical solution rather than a complex combination medical treatment.

EXFOLIATIVE GLAUCOMA

Pseudoexfoliation glaucoma (PEG) is a form of OAG where there is accumulation of exfoliation material along all the aqueous outflow pathways. Since the exfoliation material is found especially in

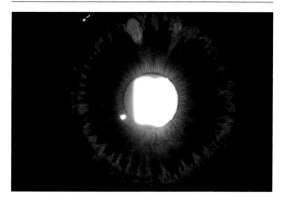

Figure 5.3 Pigmentray glaucoma: slit-like iris defects seen on transillumination.

the trabeculum and Schlemm's canal, NPGS can also be considered for this condition. For the NPGS-trained surgeon, opening Schlemm's canal in a pseudoexfoliation patient can be spectacular. Exfoliation material is found in abundance in the lumen of the canal. This material can be peeled away from the exposed trabeculum to help reestablish filtration. The IOP drops to acceptable levels for several years and when exfoliation material reaccumulates, the site of filtration can be revised to restore filtration. NPGS can be performed alone or in conjunction with cataract extraction according to the patient's age, cataract status and refractive error.

APHAKIC AND PSEUDOPHAKIC GLAUCOMA

Formerly, glaucoma specialists relied heavily on medications in order to lower IOP to acceptable levels in aphakic glaucoma. Progressive loss of visual field and eventual loss of vision were often the rule. Trabeculectomies were not considered a valid proposition because they necessitate peripheral iridectomy. In aphakic glaucoma, an iridectomy is not desirable because the vitreous may move forward through the iridectomy and block the filtration site. Tractional retinal detachment is not an uncommon complication in these combined vitrectomy–trabeculectomies, and there is a relatively high incidence of suprachoroidal hemorrhage. NPGS does not require iridectomy; therefore, it is particularly indicated in aphakic glaucoma. The only drawback of NPGS in this particular glaucoma is the status of the trabeculum. When the aphakia is longstanding, the trabeculum is often collapsed and scarred. Restoration of its function depends on its status and on the surgeon's experience and skill.

CONGENITAL AND JUVENILE GLAUCOMA

Congenital and juvenile glaucoma patients cannot rely on medications because of their long lifespan. Generally, their glaucoma is severe and results in rapid optic nerve damage and loss of vision. Initial surgical treatment is generally trabeculotomy or goniotomy. NPGS can be tried because of its low complication rate. The degree of success of NPGS is a function of the anatomic distortion of the angle structures and the surgeon's experience. NPGS will be more successful in the cases where the anatomy is less distorted. When NPGS fails, it is always possible to revert to penetrating glaucoma surgery especially in cases where the anatomy is severely distorted. Tixier and coauthors (1999) reported on NPGS in congenital glaucoma. Nine of 12 operated eyes had IOP below 16 mmHg at 10 months without medications. They concluded that NPGS is at least as effective as trabeculectomy in congenital glaucoma but it has fewer complications because the site of filtration is not perforated.

GLAUCOMA SECONDARY TO UVEITIS

When elevated IOP persists after uveitis has been controlled, glaucoma surgery is indicated. NPGS is indicated in these cases because it explores the site of resistance to aqueous outflow. During the inflammatory phases the trabeculum ultrastructure undergoes changes which interferes with normal function. These changes are mostly temporary but when they are permanent, glaucoma results. The trabeculum can be 'reconditioned' to improve filtration. However, in cases with multiple peripheral anterior synechiae NPGS may not be effective.

RELATIVE CONTRAINDICATIONS FOR NONPENETRATING GLAUCOMA SURGERY

The relative contraindications for NPGS are inherent to the status of the trabeculum because the outcome of this surgery relies on the integrity of this structure.

NARROW ANGLE GLAUCOMA

At present, many glaucomatologists consider that the treatment of choice in narrow angle glaucoma (NAG) is cataract/lens extraction. Laser iridotomy or surgical iridectomy is only a temporary measure. Removal of the crystalline lens deepens the anterior chamber and opens the angle of the eye. When NAG has persisted for some time, glaucoma surgery might be indicated in combination with lens extraction. In this case, NPGS may be attempted, even though the trabeculum might not respond to the surgery.

STATUS POST-LASER TRABECULOPLASTY

In eyes previously treated by laser trabeculoplasty, the trabeculum might be friable and may rupture during surgery. NPGS is then converted to a classical trabeculectomy.

ABSOLUTE CONTRAINDICATIONS FOR NONPENETRATING GLAUCOMA SURGERY

NEOVASCULAR GLAUCOMA

In neovascular glaucoma, new blood vessels invade the angle. NPGS will fail in these cases because the iridocorneal angle is invaded by blood vessels. The trabeculum loses its filtering function because of the presence of the neovascularization.

SURGICAL TECHNIQUES OF NONPENETRATING GLAUCOMA SURGERY

DEEP SCLERECTOMY

Usually, 3–4 ml of a solution of bupivacaine (0.75%) xylocaine (4%) and hyaluronidase (50 U) is sufficient for successful local anesthesia. Topical and subconjunctival anesthesia is also possible and has been performed successfully in selected cases. A superior rectus muscle traction suture is placed and the eyeball is rotated to expose the site of the deep sclerectomy (DS) (usually the superior quadrant). To avoid superior rectus muscle bleeding, a superior intracorneal suture may be placed, not too near the limbus so that anterior dissection of DS is not

---

Box 5.1 Surgical instruments for deep sclerectomy and viscocanalostomy

Traction sutures
Wescott scissors
Nontoothed forceps
Hockey stick
No. 11 stainless steel blade
Crescent ruby blade
15° diamond blade
Blunt forceps
10-0 nylon sutures
Collagen implant (Weck)
HEMA implants
High viscosity hyaluronic acid

---

harmed. Box 5.1 gives a list of instruments required for DS. The conjunctiva is opened either at the limbus or in the fornix. The limbal incision offers a better scleral exposition but needs more careful closure, especially when antimetabolites are used. The sclera is exposed and moderate hemostasis is performed. To facilitate the scleral dissection, all Tenon's capsule residue should be removed with a hockey stick. Sites with large aqueous drainage veins have to be avoided, to preserve as much as possible the physiological pathways of aqueous humor outflow.

A superficial scleral flap measuring 5 × 5 mm is dissected including one-third of the scleral thickness (about 300 µm) (Figure 5.4). The initial incision is done with a No.11 stainless steel blade. The horizontal dissection is done with a crescent ruby blade. To be able to later dissect the corneal stroma down to Descemet's membrane, the scleral flap is dissected 1–1.5 mm into clear cornea.

In patients with high risk of sclero-conjunctival scar formation (young, secondary glaucoma, and blacks), a sponge soaked in mitomycin-C (0.02%) may be placed for 45 seconds in the scleral bed and between the sclera and Tenon's capsule.

Deep sclero-keratectomy is done by performing a second deep scleral flap (4 × 4 mm) (Figure 5.5). The two lateral and the posterior deep scleral incisions are made using a 15° diamond blade. The deep flap is smaller than the superficial one leaving a step of sclera on the three sides. This will allow a tighter

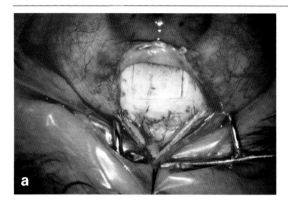 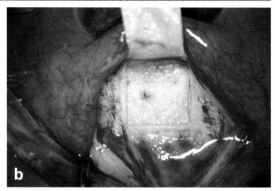

Figure 5.4 (a) Delineation of superficial scleral flap with metal blade, depth of incision about 300 μm. (b) Extension of superficial scleral flap into clear cornea for 1–1.5 mm.

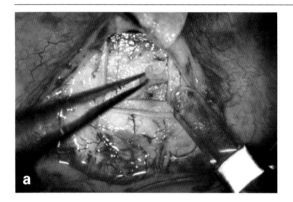 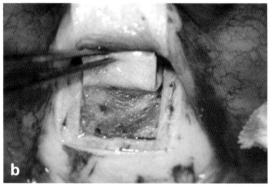

Figure 5.5 (a) Beginning of a deep sclerotomy horizontal dissection with a ruby blade. (b) Horizontal dissection in progress – halfway stage.

closure of the superficial flap in case of an intra-operative perforation of the TDM. The deep scleral flap is then dissected horizontally using the ruby blade. The remaining scleral layer should be as thin as possible (50–100 μm). Deep sclerectomy is preferably started first in the posterior part of the deep scleral flap. Reaching the anterior part of the dissection, Schlemm's canal is unroofed (Figure 5.6). Schlemm's canal is located anterior to the scleral spur where the scleral fibers are regularly oriented, parallel to the limbus. In patients with congenital glaucoma, Schlemm's canal localization is more difficult, because it is often situated more posteriorly. Schlemm's canal is opened and the sclerocorneal

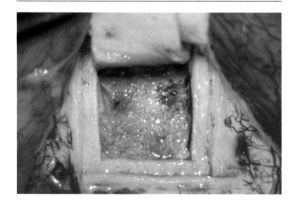

Figure 5.6 Complete opening of Schlemm's canal.

dissection is prolonged anteriorly for 1–1.5 mm to remove the sclerocorneal tissue behind the anterior trabeculum and Descemet's membrane. This step of the surgery is quite challenging because there is a high risk of perforation of the anterior chamber. The best way to perform this last dissection is to do two radial corneal cuts without touching the anterior trabeculum or Descemet's membrane. This is done with the 15° diamond knife. When the anterior dissection between the corneal stroma and Descemet's membrane is completed, the deep scleral flap is cut anteriorly using the diamond knife (Figure 5.7). At this stage, there should be a diffuse percolation of aqueous through the remaining TDM. The juxtacanalicular trabeculum and Schlemm's endothelium are then removed using a small blunt forceps (Figure 5.8). The superficial scleral flap is then closed and secured with two loose 10-0 nylon sutures. In this manner, the procedure has evolved into a combination of deep sclerectomy and ab externo trabeculectomy.

THE USE OF IMPLANTS

To avoid a secondary collapse of the superficial flap over the TDM and the remaining scleral layer, a collagen implant is placed in the scleral bed and secured with a single 10-0 nylon suture (Figure 5.9). The implant is processed from porcine scleral collagen. It increases in volume after contact with aqueous and is slowly resorbed within 6–9 months

leaving a scleral space for aqueous filtration. Other implants that can be used to fill the sclerocorneal space left after DS dissection include a reticulated hyaluronic acid implant that resorbs in about 3 months and a nonabsorbable T-shaped hydrophilic acrylic implant. The role of implants in nonpenetrating surgery is still controversial, but the bulk of studies comparing DS with an implant versus DS without, have shown higher success rates with the use of an implant.

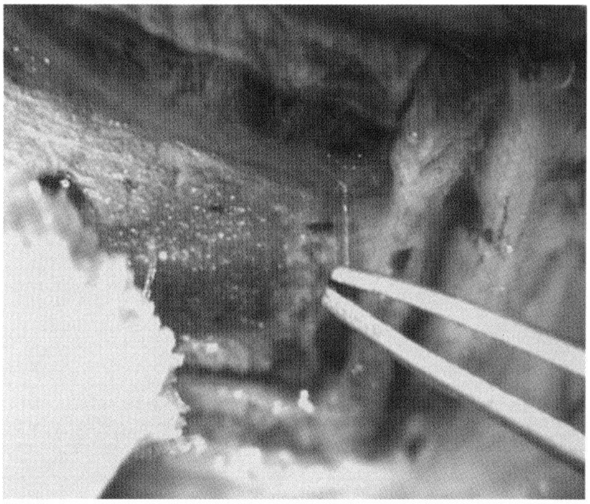

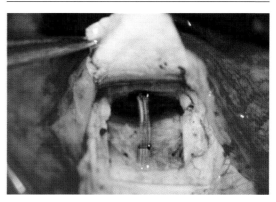

Figure 5.8 Peeling of inner endothelium of Schlemm's canal and juxtacanalicular trabeculum with the double plated forceps.

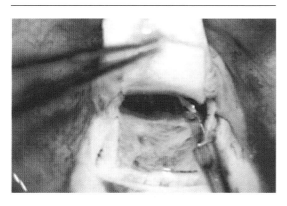

Figure 5.7 Final stage of anterior dissection of deep scleral flap by cuts with a diamond or metal blade.

Figure 5.9 Collagen implant sutured in a scleral bed. This implant will serve as a space maintainer to create an intrascleral space for aqueous humour filtration.

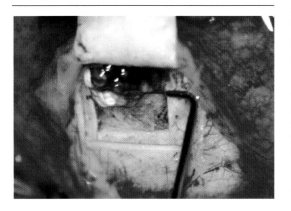

Figure 5.10 Injection of Healon GV in the scleral space.

VISCOCANALOSTOMY

In the case of viscocanalostomy, high viscosity hyaluronic acid is injected into the two surgically created ostia of Schlemm's canal, aiming at dilating both the ostia and the canal (Figure 5.10). See Box 5.1 for the list of surgical instruments. It is also placed in the scleral bed. The material is resorbed in 4–5 days. The superficial scleral flap has to be tightly sutured in order to keep the viscoelastic substance in situ and to force the aqueous percolating through the TDM into the two ostia.

ND-YAG GONIOPUNCTURE AFTER DS
(Figure 5.11)

When filtration through TDM is considered to be insufficient because of elevated IOP, Nd:YAG goniopuncture can be done. Using a gonioscopy contact lens, the aiming beam is focused on the semitransparent TDM. Using the free-running Q switched mode, with a power of 4–5 mJ, two to 15 shots are applied. This should result in the formation of microscopic holes through the TDM allowing a direct passage of aqueous from the anterior chamber to the subconjunctival space. The success rate of Nd:YAG laser goniopuncture is satisfactory,

with an immediate reduction in IOP of about 50%. The success of goniopuncture depends mainly on the thickness of the TDM, hence the importance of a sufficiently deep intraoperative dissection.

By opening the TDM, however, goniopuncture can transform a nonperforating filtration procedure into a perforating one. Although the potential risk of late bleb-related endophthalmitis may be increased after goniopuncture, no such case has been reported.

COMPLICATIONS OF NONPENETRATING SURGERY

There is an agreement among published reports that nonpenetrating surgery has a lower rate of complications when compared to conventional trabeculectomy, with or without antimetabolites. This is largely due to the eye not being fully penetrated as in trabeculectomies and aqueous percolating through the remaining TDM.

With the increase in popularity of this type of surgery, various reports have been published on specific complications that pertain to it, or occur more commonly. Complications of NPGS can be intraoperative, early postoperative or late postoperative. A comprehensive knowledge of the incidence of these complications as well as an understanding of the best ways to deal with them will help in making the correct diagnosis and subsequent management decisions.

INTRAOPERATIVE COMPLICATIONS

PERFORATION OF THE TRABECULO-DESCEMET'S MEMBRANE
Probably the commonest intraoperative complication of NPGS is perforation of the TDM. In the published reports of experienced surgeons, perforations occurred in approximately 30% of the first 10–20 cases. After the initial learning phase, a surgeon should expect a perforation in about 2–3% of cases.

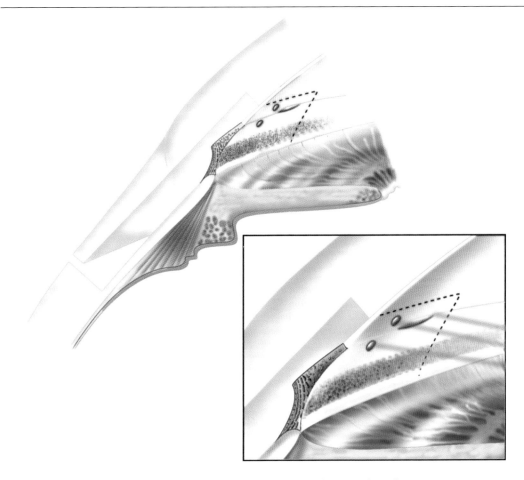

Figure 5.11 Diagram showing a laser beam creating a microscopic hole in the trabeculo-Descemet's membrane.

Types of perforation include the following:

- Transverse tears can occur at the junction of the anterior trabeculum and Descemet's membrane, probably the weakest point of the TDM, which corresponds to Schwalbe's line on gonioscopy. A perforation at this level will usually lead to the formation of a long tear, followed by immediate iris prolapse.
- TDM holes can occur during the anterior deep dissection with the knife. The holes may be small with no decrease in the depth of the ante-rior chamber (AC), or they may be large and accompanied by a shallow or flat AC, and/or iris prolapse.

MANAGEMENT OF PERFORATIONS

The two factors that determine the management of a TDM perforation are the depth of the AC, as well as the presence of iris prolapse. Small holes with no iris prolapse or loss of AC depth can be ignored and the surgery continued normally. Small or large perforations with a shallow or flat AC and no iris prolapse should be treated to prevent subsequent iris prolapse or formation of peripheral anterior synechiae. Viscoelastic material should be injected, through a paracentesis, into the AC under the TDM window. The smallest possible amount of viscoelastic material should be used to avoid a postoperative IOP spike. In addition, an implant resting on the perforation site may help tamponade the hole. The superficial scleral flap should be tightly sutured with six to eight 10-0 nylon sutures. If there is iris prolapse accompanying a long tear or large hole, a peripheral iridectomy needs to be done. The superficial flap should be tightly closed and viscoelastic material should be injected in the surgically created scleral space to increase outflow resistance.

Any perforation of the TDM during deep sclerectomy transforms the nonpenetrating filtering surgery into a penetrating one. Because the scleral space left after deep sclerectomy decreases the resistance to aqueous humor outflow, a very tight superficial scleral flap closure is needed.

In a series of 20 patients who underwent an intraoperative perforation of the TDM, Sanchez and colleagues reported an increased incidence of early postoperative complications such as flat AC, hypotony, choroidal detachment, inflammation, and hyphema compared with classical trabeculectomy. In this series, however, the superficial scleral flap was not tightly closed. In our experience, by closing the scleral flap with six to eight 10-0 nylon sutures, especially if done in combination with viscoelastics under the scleral flap, hypotony-related complications can be avoided in most of the cases.

HEMORRHAGES

Intraoperative hemorrhage may occur either at the conjunctival–scleral level or in the uveal tissue. It can also be seen secondary to blood reflux from Schlemm's canal ostia. Both blood and cautery-induced thermal injury may stimulate fibroblast proliferation and decrease the chances of filtration bleb survival. During the conjunctival and scleral dissections, major bleeding should be treated with light cauterization. Wet-field cautery is probably the safest tool and allows minimal scleral burns.

Strong topical vasoconstrictors may help minimize the need for cautery.

Intraocular bleeding is rare and may originate from uveal or retinal vessels; it usually occurs because of decreased IOP. NPGS lowers the incidence of this complication because the IOP drop is slower than it is during trabeculectomy. However, in patients with fragile vessels, arterial hypertension and/or anticoagulation therapy, intraocular bleeding may still occur especially if the preoperative IOP is exceedingly high. While small iris hemorrhages are insignificant, major retinal or choroidal bleeding may be sight threatening.

Blood reflux from Schlemm's canal ostia may occur when the episcleral venous pressure is higher than the IOP. This complication makes dissection of TDM difficult. Blood reflux may be stopped by injecting high molecular weight viscoelastic into both Schlemm's canal ostia by a special cannula (Alcon Grieshaber AG, Schaffhausen, Switzerland), or by injecting a balanced salt solution into the anterior chamber, thereby increasing the IOP. This reflux may also occur after surgery during Valsalva episodes.

EARLY POSTOPERATIVE COMPLICATIONS

WOUND LEAK

Wound leak or positive Seidel test occurs with the same frequency after trabeculectomy and NPGS, as it is almost always due to inadequate wound closure. In most cases the wound leak closes after discontinuation of steroid therapy. Rarely, a surgical intervention is necessary to repair it.

HYPHEMA

Hyphema is a rare complication after NPGS. The blood in the anterior chamber may originate either from a rupture of a small iris vessel such as in Fuchs heterochromia (Amsler sign), or from a leak of red blood cells through the TDM, usually through microperforations. Usually the erythrocytes are diffusely present within the anterior chamber. No particular treatment is needed in this situation, and the anterior chamber clears itself within a few days with routinely prescribed topical anti-inflammatory treatment.

INFLAMMATION

The degree of inflammatory reaction following surgical trauma is considerably less in NPGS compared to trabeculectomy. This is mainly due to the fact that the anterior chamber is not penetrated, and that an iridectomy is not necessary.

HYPOTONY

The mean IOP after nonpenetrating filtering surgeries has been reported to be around 5 mmHg on the first postoperative day. Fifty percent of the patients present with early ocular hypotony. If it is short lived and is not associated with any secondary complications, ocular hypotony should not cause worry. In our experience, even an IOP of 0–2 mmHg on the first postoperative day does not need specific treatment. Early hypotony without any perforation is an excellent indicator of good surgical dissection. According to experimental work on the outflow resistance of the TDM, the immediate postoperative IOP should be very low since the outflow facility after a deep sclerectomy is about 130 times higher. Because the TDM offers enough resistance to avoid AC collapse; a flat AC has not been reported after NPGS.

POSTOPERATIVE INCREASE IN IOP

Postoperative increases in IOP, secondary to the superficial scleral flap being closed too tightly, are often observed after trabeculectomy and needs either laser suture lysis and/or ocular massage, unless releasable sutures were used. Because the main site of postoperative aqueous humor outflow resistance after NPGS is located at the TDM level, this complication should not occur if the dissection of the membrane has been done properly. Early postoperative IOP spikes occur rarely and can be due to the following:

* insufficient surgical dissection, most common after nonpenetrating filtering surgeries by inexperienced surgeons

* hemorrhage in the scleral bed, which usually spontaneously resorbs within a few days
* excess viscoelastic remaining in the AC, mainly after combined surgeries or of the AC reformation following perforation of the TDM
* malignant glaucoma
* postoperative rupture of the TDM with iris prolapse, secondary to increased IOP from rubbing the eye or a Valsalva maneuver
* peripheral anterior synechia formation at the site of the filtering window, often secondary to an intraoperative microperforation
* steroid induced IOP spike within the first postoperative weeks.

LATE POSTOPERATIVE COMPLICATIONS

Unlike immediate postoperative complications, late postoperative complications occur with the same frequency in penetrating glaucoma surgery and NPGS. This may be explained by the fact that late complications are often related to excessive scarring of the operated tissues and that the surgical procedure as such does not influence this process.

LATE RUPTURE OF THE TRABECULO-DESCEMET'S MEMBRANE

The risk of membrane rupture decreases with time because the post-membrane outflow resistance slowly increases for several weeks after surgery. However, rupture can occur after severe ocular trauma. Often there is a concomitant iris prolapse with a distorted pupil and darkening of the subconjunctival area. If the IOP remains under control, no further treatment is needed. However, if the iris prolapse blocks the aqueous humor outflow and the IOP rises, medical or surgical therapy should be considered.

DETACHMENT OF DESCEMET'S MEMBRANE

Detachment of Descemet's membrane is a rare complication after NPGS. We estimate it to occur in one out of 250–300 operated eyes. The pathogenesis depends on the type of surgery, although there appears to be an anatomic predisposition in some patients. With viscocanalostomy, detachment is related to viscoelastic injection into artificial ostia of Schlemm's canal. It could be that the cannula was slightly misdirected. The detachment is noticed during the procedure or shortly afterwards. After other NPGS, this complication may be explained by the passage of aqueous humor from the scleral space into the sub-Descemet space at the anterior edge of the Descemet's window, secondary to increased intrableb pressures which may occur after trauma, development of an encysted bleb, of vigorous ocular massage. Detachment of Descemet's membrane is usually diagnosed 4–8 weeks postoperatively. After viscocanalostomy, the cornea associated with the Descemet's detachment remains clear probably because of the intact endothelium–Descemet's complex and the chemical properties of sodium hyaluronate. Patients complain of decreased visual acuity if the detachment extends over the visual axis because of adjacent corneal edema. Blood may also be seen in the retro-Descemet's space.

Whether or not patients have the detachment repaired, the final visual acuities are similar to the preoperative acuity. In addition there is excellent IOP control. The detachment usually reattaches spontaneously after treatment of causative factors such as high intrableb pressure.

PERIPHERAL ANTERIOR SYNECHIA

The iris may adhere to the trabeculo-Descemet's window and form peripheral anterior synechia (PAS) due to intraoperative microperforation with microiris prolapse, iris entrapment into a goniopuncture hole, which usually occurs rapidly after laser treatment, or rupture of the TDM (e.g. blunt trauma) with subsequent iris prolapse. There may be an associated increase in IOP if there is insufficient aqueous humor flow through the membrane. Laser burns may be used to shrink the iris away from the Descemet's window. If this fails, medical or secondary surgical treatment should be considered.

SCLERAL ECTASIA

In the literature there is a single reported case of scleral ectasia following deep sclerectomy in a 12-year-old girl with chronic arthritis and uveitis complicated with glaucoma. Rare as it is, this complication should be considered in patients with high myopia, or chronic uveitis. The use of antimetabolites intra- or postoperatively may also increase the risk of this complication.

MECHANISMS OF FILTRATION AFTER NONPENETRATING GLAUCOMA SURGERY

Aqueous humor flow through TDM and aqueous resorption after its passage through TDM help distinguish NPGS from trabeculectomy.

FLOW THROUGH THE TRABECULO–DESCEMET'S MEMBRANE

The TDM offers resistance to aqueous outflow. This resistance will provide a slow decrease in IOP during surgery and will account for the reliable and reproducible IOP on the first postoperative day. Thus, the main advantage of the TDM is to reduce immediate postoperative complications such as hypotony, flat anterior chambers, choroidal detachments, and/or cataracts.

In a study of enucleated human eyes unsuitable for keratoplasty, the mean decrease in IOP during NPGS was 2.7 ± 0.6 mmHg/min. TDM resistance decreased from a mean of 5.34 ± 0.19 ml/min/mmHg to a mean of 0.41 ± 0.16 ml/min/mmHg. A resistance of 0.41 ± 0.16 ml/min/mmHg is apparently low enough to ensure a low IOP but high enough to maintain the AC depth and to avoid postoperative complications of hypotony. In the same study, Dr Rossier and coauthors histologically examined the surgical site using ocular perfusion with ferritin. They were able to demonstrate that the main outflow through TDM occurred at the level of the anterior trabeculum. There was also some outflow through the posterior trabeculum and Descemet's membrane.

AQUEOUS HUMOR RESORPTION

After the passage of aqueous humor through the TDM, there are four possible ways in which aqueous humor resorption may occur: through the subconjunctival bleb, through the intrascleral bleb, through the subchoroidal space, and through Schlemm's canal.

SUBCONJUNCTIVAL BLEB

As after trabeculectomy, patients undergoing NPGS have, in almost 100% of the cases, a diffuse, subconjunctival bleb on the first postoperative day. Years after the operation, all successful cases still showed a low profile and diffuse subconjunctival filtering bleb with ultrasound biomicroscopy (UBM). This bleb is usually smaller than the one seen after trabeculectomy.

INTRASCLERAL BLEB

When the deep sclerectomy is performed, a volume of sclera ranging between 5 and 8 mm^3 is removed. If the superficial scleral flap does not collapse, this scleral volume may be transformed into an intrascleral filtering bleb. In order to keep this intrascleral volume, different implants may be used, such as the collagen implant. Hyaluronic acid or nonresorbable HEMA implants have also been used. An intrascleral bleb was observed in more than 90% of the cases with UBM. The mean volume of the intrascleral bleb was 1.8 mm^3 (Kazakova D et al. Ultrasound biomicroscopic study: long term results after deep sclerectomy. Unpublished data). In the intrascleral filtering bleb, the aqueous resorption may be different from that occurring in the subconjunctival bleb. The aqueous is probably resorbed by new aqueous drainage vessels as demonstrated in a study on rabbits by Delarive and coworkers (Delarive T et al. Deep sclerectomy with collagen implant: an animal model. Unpublished data). Similar results were obtained by Nguyen and coworkers using the same model and performing anterior segment fluorescein and indocyanin green angiography (Nguyen C et al. Aqueous drainage veins formation after deep sclerectomy with and without collagen implant using fluorescein and indocyanin green anterior segment angiography. Unpublished data).

SUBCHOROIDAL SPACE

Since the remaining layer of sclera over the ciliary body and peripheral choroid after deep sclerectomy is very thin, there may be drainage of aqueous humor into the suprachoroidal space. Using UBM, it is possible to observe fluid between the ciliary body and the remaining sclera in 45% of the patients studied years after deep sclerectomy (Kazakova D et al. Unpublished data). Aqueous in the choroidal space may indicate increased uveoscleral outflow, or it could indicate a chronic ciliary body detachment with reduced aqueous production.

SCHLEMM'S CANAL

When performing the deep sclerectomy dissection, Schlemm's canal is opened and unroofed. On either side of the deep sclerectomy the two ostia of Schlemm's canal may drain the aqueous humor into the episcleral veins. This mechanism may be more important after viscocanalostomy since the Schlemm's canal is dilated with high viscosity hyaluronic acid during the surgery. It may also play a role when an HEMA implant is used since this implant has two arms inserted into the two ostia of Schlemm's canal.

DOES NONPENETRATING GLAUCOMA SURGERY LOWER THE INTRAOCULAR PRESSURE?

In a prospective, nonrandomized trial, Mermoud and co-workers in 1999 compared 44 patients with medically uncontrolled primary open angle glaucoma who underwent deep sclerectomy with collagen implant with a matched group of 44 patients who underwent trabeculectomy. Complete success at 24 months postoperatively, defined as an IOP lower than 21 mmHg without medications, was 69% in the deep sclerectomy group versus 57% in the trabeculectomy group. When considering the patients needing laser goniopuncture as failed cases, the complete success rate of deep sclerectomy with collagen implant was 66%. In another non-randomized, prospective clinical trial, 100 eyes of 100 consecutive patients with medically uncontrolled primary and secondary open angle glaucoma underwent deep sclerectomy with collagen implant. The rate of complete success at 36 months postoperatively, defined as an IOP lower than 21 mmHg without medications, was 44.6%. Qualified success at 36 months postoperatively, defined as an IOP lower than 21 mmHg with and without medication, was 97.7%. There was no difference in reduction of IOP, number of patients requiring antiglaucoma medications, or success rates for the different types of open angle glaucoma. There was, however, a tendency for lower success rates in patients with pseudoexfoliative and pseudophakic glaucoma. In a recent study, Shaarawy and coworkers reported that the mean IOP of 105 patients who underwent deep sclerectomy with a collagen implant was 11.8 mmHg after 5 years; 63% had complete success and 95.1% had qualified success.

CONCLUSION

When performed by different investigators, NPGS results in a significant decrease in IOP along with a reasonable success rate after several years of follow-up. The immediate postoperative complication rates are low, and visual acuity is relatively unaffected postoperatively. This is mainly due to the presence of the TDM, which allows a progressive drop in IOP and offers enough resistance to reduce immediate postoperative complications. Additional randomized clinical trials comparing this procedure to trabulectomy are needed.

FURTHER READING

Bas JM, Goethals MJ. Non-penetrating deep sclerectomy preliminary results. Bull Soc Belge Ophtalmol 1999; 272: 55–9.

Bellows AR, Chylack LT Jr, Epstein DL, Hutchinson BT. Choroidal effusion during glaucoma surgery in patients with prominent episcleral vessels. Arch Ophthalmol 1979; 97: 493–7.

Bellows AR, Chylack LT Jr, Hutchinson BT. Choroidal detachment. Clinical manifestation, therapy and mechanism of formation. Ophthalmology 1981; 88: 1107–15.

Bylsma S. Nonpenetrating deep sclerectomy: collagen implant and viscocanalostomy procedures. Int Ophthalmol Clin 1999; 39: 103–19.

Carassa R. Viscocanalaostomy versus trabeculectomy: a 12 months prospective randomized study. Boston, USA. 2000.

Chiou AG, Mermoud A, Jewelewicz DA. Post-operative inflammation following deep sclerectomy with collagen implant versus standard trabeculectomy. Graefes Arch Clin Exp Ophthalmol 1998; 236: 593–6.

Dahan E, Drusedau MU. Nonpenetrating filtration surgery for glaucoma: control by surgery only. J Cataract Refract Surg 2000; 26: 695–701.

Demailly P, Jeanteur-Lunel MN, Berkani M et al. [Non-penetrating deep sclerectomy combined with a collagen implant in primary open-angle glaucoma. Medium-term retrospective results]. J Fr Ophtalmol 1996; 19: 659–66.

El Sayyad F, Helal M, El-Kholify H, Khalil M, El-Maghraby A. Nonpenetrating deep sclerectomy versus trabeculectomy in bilateral primary open-angle glaucoma. Ophthalmology 2000; 107: 1671–4.

Fedorov SN, Ioffe DI, Ronkina TI. [Glaucoma surgery—deep sclerectomy]. Vestn Oftalmol 1982; 4: 6–10.

Gianoli F, Schnyder CC, Bovey E, Mermoud A. Combined surgery for cataract and glaucoma: phacoemulsification and deep sclerectomy compared with phacoemulsification and trabeculectomy [see comments]. J Cataract Refract Surg 1999; 25: 340–6.

Gimbel HV, Penno EE, Ferensowicz M. Combined cataract surgery, intraocular lens implantation, and viscocanalostomy. J Cataract Refract Surg 1999; 25: 1370–5.

Hamel M, Shaarawy T, Mermoud, A. Deep sclerectomy with collagen implant in glaucomatous patients with high myopia. J Cataract Refract Surg 2001; 27: 1410–17.

Jay JL, Allan D. The benefit of early trabeculectomy versus conventional management in primary open angle glaucoma relative to severity of disease. Eye 1989; 3: 528–35.

Karlen ME, Sanchez E, Schnyder CC, Sickenberg M, Mermoud A. Deep sclerectomy with collagen implant: medium term results [See comments]. Br J Ophthalmol 1999; 83: 6–11.

Kozlov VI, Bagrov SN, Anisimova SY, Osipov AV, Mogilevtsev VV. Nonpenetrating deep sclerectomy with collagen. Eye Microsurg (Russian) 1990; 3: 157–62.

Lavin MJ, Wormald RP, Migdal CS, Hitchings RA. The influence of prior therapy on the success of trabeculectomy. Arch Ophthalmol 1990; 108: 1543–8.

Massy J, Gruber D, Muraine M, Brasseur G. [Non-penetrating deep sclerectomy in the surgical treatment of chronic open-angle glaucoma. Mid-term results]. J Fr Ophtalmol 1999; 22: 292–8.

Mermoud A. Sinusotomy and deep sclerectomy. Eye 2000; 14: 531–5.

Mermoud A, Schnyder CC, Sickenberg M et al. Comparison of deep sclerectomy with collagen implant and trabeculectomy in open-angle glaucoma [See comments]. J Cataract Refract Surg 1999; 25: 323–31.

Mitchell P, Hourihan F, Sandbach J, Wang JJ. The relationship between glaucoma and myopia: the Blue Mountains Eye Study [See comments]. Ophthalmology 1999; 106: 2010–15.

Nguyen C, Shaarawy T. Experimental studies in non-penetrating glaucoma surgery. In: Mermoud A, Shaarawy T, eds. Non-penetrating glaucoma surgery. London: Martin Dunitz, 2001: 67–86.

Ruderman JM, Harbin TS Jr, Campbell DG. Postoperative suprachoroidal hemorrhage following filtration procedures. Arch Ophthalmol 1986; 104: 201–5.

Sanchez E, Schnyder CC, Sickenberg M et al. Deep sclerectomy: results with and without collagen implant. Int Ophthalmol 1996; 20: 157–62.

Sanchez E, Schnyder CC, Mermoud A. [Comparative results of deep sclerectomy transformed to trabeculectomy and classical trabeculectomy]. Klin Monatsbl Augenheilkd 1997; 210: 261–4.

Shaarawy T, Mermoud A. Long term results of deep sclerectomy with collagen implant in pseudoexfoliative glaucoma. Ophthal Res 2000; 32.

Shaarawy T, Karlen ME, Sanchez E et al. Five-year results of deep sclerectomy with collagen implant. J Cataract Refract Surg 2001; 27: 1770–8.

Shaarawy T, Nguyen C, Achache F, Schnyder CC, Mermoud A. Long-term results of viscocanalostomy in Caucasians. AAO, Dallas, USA, 2000.

Shaarawy T, Schnyder CC, Nguyen C, Mermoud A. Long-term results of deep sclerectomy with collagen implant in pseudophakic glaucoma patients. AAO, Dallas, USA, 2000.

Shaarawy T, Nguyen C, Achache F, Schnyder CC, Mermoud A. Deep sclerectomy with and without collagen implant: Long-term prospective study. Mermoud A and Shaarawy T 2001. Lausanne, Switzerland.

Sourdille P, Santiago PY, Villain F et al. Reticulated hyaluronic acid implant in nonperforating trabecular surgery [See comments]. J Cataract Refract Surg 1999; 25: 332–9.

Stegmann R, Pienaar A, Miller D. Viscocanalostomy for open-angle glaucoma in black African patients. J Cataract Refract Surg 1999; 25: 316–22.

Tixier J, Dureau P, Becquet F, Dufier JL. [Deep sclerectomy in congenital glaucoma. Preliminary results]. J Fr Ophtalmol 1999; 22: 545–8.

6. One-site combined cataract and glaucoma surgery

Paul Palmberg and Kyoko Ishida

ONE-SITE VERSUS TWO-SITE COMBINED PROCEDURES

There has been considerable controversy about whether combined procedures should be done with a two-site technique (temporal clear cornea phacoemulsification and superior site trabeculectomy) or through a one-site incision above. Claims that a two-site approach yields better glaucoma control than a one-site approach have been made on the basis of small studies utilizing quite different techniques and often without the aid of mitomycin-C. In a comprehensive review, Jampel and co-workers (2002) concluded that there was moderately strong evidence that mitomycin-C augmentation yielded better IOP control (2–4 mmHg difference), but only weak evidence that two-site procedures pro-

vided better control than one-site procedures (1–3 mmHg) or that phacoemulsification gave better results than nuclear expression techniques (1–3 mmHg).

Our long-term results for one-site combined procedures performed with a high dose of mitomycin-C indicate, however, that one does not need to use a two-site procedure to obtain optimal glaucoma control (Tables 6.1 and 6.2, Figures 6.1 and 6.2), and that there was no difference between the IOP control obtained with combined procedures utilizing phacoemulsification versus extracapsular cataract extraction.

The genuine advantages of a two-site procedure all have to do with the performance of the cataract operation. A two-site approach allows a surgeon who performs a lot of clear cornea cataract surgery

Table 6.1 Combined cataract and glaucoma filtering surgery: pressure control and visual field data

	IOP (mmHg)	IOP sample size (No)	MD (dB)	ChMD	PSD (dB)	ChPSD	HVF sample size (No)
Pre-op	23.2	265	−13.1		5.19		226
1 day	11.1						
1 week	9.6						
1 month	9.6						
3 months	10.2						
6 months	10.6						
1 year	11.2	226	−9.2	2.9	5.16	0.04	144
2 years	11.1	193	−9.1	3.2	5.2	−0.13	115
3 years	10.9	168	−8.4	3.5	4.89	0.04	98
4 years	10.8	151	−8.9	3.9	5.2	−0.19	89
5 years	10.8	136	−8	3.4	5.22	−0.83	76
6 years	11.2	102	−7.7	3.4	5.43	−0.62	57
7 years	10.3	82	−8.2	3.7	5.53	−0.25	47
8 years	11.3	67	−8.4	3.4	5.63	−0.42	34
9 years	9.9	41	−8.2	4.6	6.43	−1.81	21
10 years	10.3	26	−9.9	5.9	6.97	−1.43	10

IOP, intraocular pressure; No., number; MD, mean deviation; ChMD, change in mean deviation; PSD, patter standard deviation; ChPSD, change in pattern standard deviation; HVF, Humphery visual field.

Table 6.2 Life table analysis of the cumulative survival rate for IOP control without medication or reoperation

Months	IOP <21 mmHg	No.	IOP <16 mmHg	No.
12	97.6%	218	77.1%	172
24	95.3%	196	69.5%	143
60	91.4%	106	62.2%	71
84	86.3%	59	54.1%	35
120	84.0%	8	51.0%	4

IOP, intraocular pressure; No., number.

and only a few trabeculectomies or combined procedures to perform the cataract surgery they do best. Furthermore, a temporal approach allows one to obtain an optimal red reflex (and to avoid pooling of fluid) by simply tilting the patient's head slightly to the side, rather than having to hyperextend the neck as when working above. In patients with deep-set eyes, a temporal approach avoids having to work over a prominent brow, which might reduce the range of motion of the phaco instrument. In patients with narrow palpebral fissures, a temporal approach yields adequate visualization of the phacoemulsification tip during its

excursion in sculpting a groove in the lens nucleus. In the shallow anterior chamber of angle closure patients, the more anterior entry of a temporal clear corneal wound allows one to use a more vertical approach to the lens that reduces the risk of touching and injuring the iris with the phacoemulsification tip. On the other hand, when working at the superior limbus, if one does not convert the phacoemulsification tunnel into the filter, one would have the additional difficulty of performing phacoemulsification under a scleral flap.

For all these reasons having to do with better performance of the cataract portion of the operation, we have in fact chosen to do two-site procedures for the past few years. However, for those preferring one-site phacoemulsification combined procedures at the superior limbus, or those having only the equipment to perform extracapsular combined procedures, our prior experience shows that the outcome of the glaucoma portion of the procedure is not inferior.

In favor of combined procedures in which a phacoemulsification tunnel above is converted into a filter, the use of a single site saves time, as only one wound has to be made and the microscope does not need to be repositioned to move from one site to another.

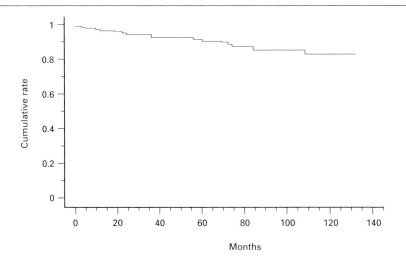

Figure 6.1 The cumulative survival rate (life table analysis) for maintenance of intraocular pressure <21 mmHg on all annual visits, without need for supplemental medical therapy or reoperation.

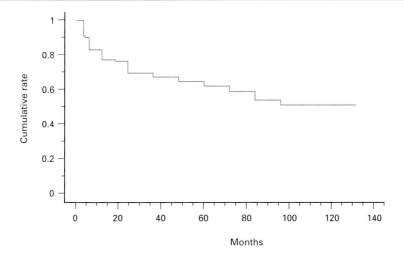

Figure 6.2 The cumulative survival rate (life table analysis) for maintenance of intraocular pressure <16 mmHg on all annual visits, without need for supplemental medical therapy or reoperation.

RESULTS OF OUR ONE-SITE COMBINED PROCEDURES WITH MITOMYCIN C

From April 1991 through December 1995 we performed 265 combined cataract (extracapsular or phacoemulsification) and glaucoma filtering procedures with mitomycin C. We asked all of the patients to return at least annually so that we could monitor their course. With the approval of the Institutional Review Board we retrospectively review the data from time to time. We presently have 5-year follow-up data for only half of the subjects. On the basis of phone calls and letters sent to patients and referring physicians, and Social Security lists of those who are deceased, we attribute the loss to follow-up primarily to changes in insurance status, and, to a lesser extent, to patients moving away, living in foreign countries, or passing away.

We were able to perform Humphrey visual field testing with reliable results on 226 eyes (85.3%). Subjects who could not perform Humphrey visual field testing were followed with Goldmann kinetic perimetry, which we have not tried to quantitate. The pressure control and visual field data are pre-

sented in Tables 6.1 and 6.2 and Figures 6.1 and 6.2. The IOP fell from a mean preoperative value of 23.2 mmHg to a mean of 11.1 mmHg on day 1, showing that my technique for intraoperative adjustment of the scleral resistance to yield a pressure of 8–12 mmHg at equilibrium flow was successful. The mean IOP during the 10 years of follow-up ranged from 9.9 to 11.3 mmHg, indicating that the strategy of using mitomycin C to retard the formation of additional resistance to flow was successful. The pressures shown in Table 6.1 are those obtained on annual visits, whether or not medication was added or interventions were performed (argon laser suture lysis, YAG laser treatment of the internal filtration ostium, needling of the scleral tunnel and/or bleb, or reoperation). In Table 6.2, a life table analysis is given for the cumulative survival rate of control of IOP at <21 mmHg and IOP <16 mmHg without the need for medication or reoperation. The 5-year success rate for an IOP <21 mmHg was 91.4% and for a IOP <16 mmHg was 62.2%. The mean pressure was slightly lower with extracapsular combined procedures, but the success rates, average pressures at each year of follow-up, and visual field results were nearly

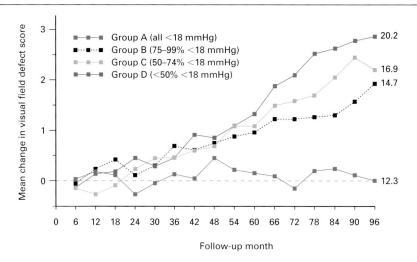

Figure 6.3 The visual field outcomes of four groups in the Advanced Glaucoma Intervention Study (AGIS). The results are plotted in months along the x-axis and in AGIS visual field units along the y-axis. The mean baseline field defect for the pooled subjects was 8.4 AGIS units, which corresponded to a mean deviation on Humphrey visual field testing of 10.5 dB. In Group A, the intraocular pressure (IOP) at all visits (over the first 6 years) was <18 mmHg, and the average IOP was 12.3 mmHg. There was no net visual field loss in 8 years of follow-up. In Group B, the IOP at 75–99% of visits was <18 mmHg, and the average IOP was 14.7 mmHg. The visual field loss averaged 1.9 AGIS units. In Group C, the IOP at 50–74% of visits was <18 mmHg, and the average IOP was 16.9 mmHg. The visual field loss averaged 2.2 AGIS units. In group D, the IOP at <50% of visits was <18 mmHg, and the average IOP was 20.2 mmHg. The visual field loss averaged 2.9 AGIS units. (From the AGIS Investigators. Am J Ophthalmol 2000; 130: 429–40.)

identical for extracapsular and phacoemulsification combined procedures, and so the results were pooled.

The mean value of the mean deviation (MD) pre-operatively was −13.1 dB. The MD was improved by removal of the cataract, with the mean change in mean deviation (ChMD) from baseline values at 1 year being 2.92 ± 3.52 (SD) dB. Thereafter, the MD and ChMD did not change significantly. The preoperative pattern standard deviation (PSD) was 5.19 dB, and was unchanged by removal of the cataract. Thereafter, the PSD and the change from baseline values in PSD (ChPSD) did not change significantly.

It is noteworthy that the MD in our subjects after removal of the cataract, −9.2 dB, is similar to the baseline value of −10.5 dB reported in the Advanced Glaucoma Intervention Study (AGIS). In that study, subjects in whom the IOP after intervention was always <18 mmHg (mean IOP 12.3 mmHg) at follow-up visits did not suffer any net progression of visual field loss in 8 years, whereas those in whom the IOP was 18 mmHg or more on 1–25% of the follow-up visits (mean IOP 14.7 mmHg), 26–50% of the follow-up visits (mean IOP 16.9 mmHg) and >50% of the follow-up visits (mean IOP 20.2 mmHg) had progressively more and statistically significant visual field progression (Figure 6.3). We have argued that the AGIS results, and our previous similar results for primary filtering surgery with either 5-fluorouracil or mitomycin C, favor seeking target pressures in the low–normal range in patients with moderate-to-severe glaucoma damage. In the present study of combined filtering surgery, IOP control similar to the best group in AGIS was achieved and resulted in a similar stabilization of visual fields.

TECHNIQUE OF ONE-SITE PHACO TUNNEL FILTERING SURGERY

OVERALL STRATEGY

In the pre-antimetabolite era, filtering surgery was usually performed either superior temporally or superior nasally, to allow for repeat surgery in the other superior quadrant if needed, and to take advantage of the fact that the Tenon's capsule is thinner to each side than it is at 12 o'clock. In addition, when large (4 × 4 mm) scleral flaps were used, non-12 o'clock locations avoided cutting the anterior ciliary vessels coming down from the superior rectus. However, with the use of antimetabolites and short, tunneled incisions, our preferred site for filtration is at or very near to 12 o'clock. The intention is to create filtering blebs that even with a large surface area will be completely covered by the upper lid, to reduce the risk of bleb discomfort, leaks, and infection. To operate at that location, the surgeon and microscope are positioned about 15° off to one side of the patient's head, so as to allow comfortable access to the 12 o'clock location with the surgeon's dominant hand.

THE CONJUNCTIVAL FLAP

A fornix-based conjunctival flap was used since it gives better exposure for cataract surgery, allows easier conversion to an extracapsular procedure, and is constructed and closed more rapidly than a limbus-based flap. Despite the use of mitomycin C, early postoperative leaks were rare and all were successfully repaired.

The conjunctival flap is initiated with a 2-mm radial relaxing incision at the temporal limbus using Westcott scissors (Box 6.1). Care is taken to make sure that the dissection reaches bare sclera. The 180° superior peritomy is then fashioned 1–2 clock hours at a time. In each portion, the blunt tips of the closed scissors are first swept behind the insertion of Tenon's capsule and brought forward to the insertion (generally 1 mm behind the conjunctival insertion). Then, while the leading edge of the flap is elevated with nontoothed forceps, one

---

Box 6.1 Surgical instruments

Lid speculum
Westcott scissors
Nontoothed forceps
Cautery
Calipers
Miniblade
Crescent blade
0.12 toothed forceps
Viscoelastic
Balanced saline solution
2.7 or 3.0 keratome
Cyclodialysis spatula
2 Kuglen hooks (Storz, St Lows, MO)
Vannas scissors
Grieshaber flexible hooks
Indocyanine green
Cystotome
Utratta forceps
27 and 30-gauge cannulas
3 ml syringe
Drysdale spatula
Acrylic or silicone intraocular lens
Mitomycin C (Mutamycin, Bristol-Myers, Evanville, IN)
Acetylcholine (Miochol, Ciba Vision, Atlanta, GA)
Kelly Descemet's punch (Storz, St Louis, MO)
Cellulose spear sponges
10-0 nylon suture

---

blade of the scissors is placed behind the Tenon's insertion, and the Tenon's capsule and overlying conjunctiva are then sheared from their insertions (Figure 6.4). Care is taken to avoid making any radial dehiscence in Tenon's capsule other than at 3 and 9 o'clock. This is essential, because an intact Tenon's capsule with overlying conjunctiva will form a watertight belt when stretched tightly along the limbus at the end of the procedure.

SCLERAL WOUND CONSTRUCTION

After light cautery is applied to the intended site of filtration at 12 o'clock, any episcleral tissue is removed by elevating it with 0.12 forceps and cutting it off with a miniblade, leaving bare sclera. Any residual episcleral tissue could otherwise prevent the rotation of suture knots under the surface later on, or might proliferate postoperatively to form a fibrous cap over the filter site.

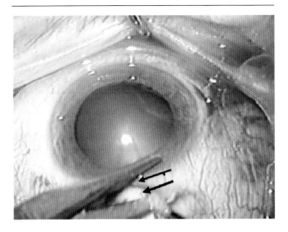

Figure 6.4 The figure illustrates the technique for cutting the Tenon's capsule (thicker arrow) and the conjunctiva (thinner arrow) at their insertions, using Westcott scissors.

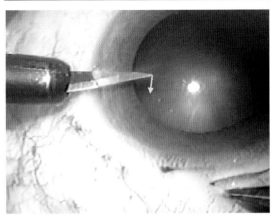

Figure 6.6 A paracentesis is begun with a miniblade at the temporal limbus. After entering the anterior chamber with the dull side of the blade held perpendicular to the limbus, the knife will be pivoted within the wound in the direction indicated by the arrow, so as to make the internal entry as wide as the external entry.

The intended 3-mm incision line is marked with calipers 1-mm behind and parallel to the limbus, at or near to 12 o'clock (Figure 6.5). The incision is then cut with a miniblade. The anterior edge of the incision is elevated with 0.12 forceps, and a crescent blade is used to create a tunnel extending 1 mm into clear cornea. A paracentesis is performed for the second port entry 2 clock hours from the scle-

ral tunnel. The miniblade is pivoted (Figure 6.6) slightly during formation of the paracentesis to yield an internal opening as wide or wider than the external opening, so that subsequent entry of the second instrument will be facilitated without compromising the watertightness of the paracentesis, and to avoid optical distortion produced by bending the cornea with movement of second instruments. The anterior chamber fluid is then replaced with a viscoelastic agent and the phacoemulsification wound is completed by entry with a 2.7- or 3.0-mm keratome (Figure 6.7).

PUPIL EXPANSION, CAPSULORHEXIS, HYDRODISSECTION, AND NUCLEUS ROTATION

It may be necessary to lyse posterior synechiae (especially in eyes that have undergone laser iridotomy or those that have been on pilocarpine), and to mechanically expand the pupil if pharmacologic dilatation proves insufficient. A cyclodialysis spatula is passed into the eye through the keratome incision and passed under the iris in an area free of posterior synechiae. It is then used to gently lift the adjacent iris in each direction for about 3 clock

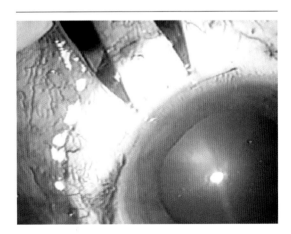

Figure 6.5 Calipers are used to mark the sclera for a 3-mm incision, placed 1 mm behind the limbus in the 12 o'clock position. The surgeon and camera are rotated 15° clockwise so that the surgeon's dominant hand is centered on the incision.

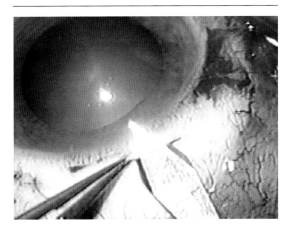

Figure 6.7 A 2.7-mm keratome is used to enter the anterior chamber at 12 o'clock.

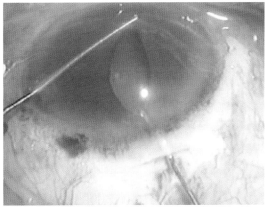

Figure 6.8 In a case with a small pupil due to long-term use of pilocarpine, the pupil is stretched vertically, using two Kuglen hooks to first capture and elevate, and then to stretch the pupil, in the technique introduced by Luther Frye.

hours, breaking any posterior synechiae encountered. The instrument should move under the iris like 'a mouse under a rug', so as avoid breaking the anterior capsule. The spatula is then brought in through the second port and often through an additional paracentesis in temporal or inferior cornea to free the remainder of the pupil margin. A small amount of viscoelastic injected behind the iris will help avoid injury to the lens capsule.

If the pupil diameter is still insufficient, the pupil can be stretched with two Kuglen hooks (Storz, St Louis, MO). These are introduced through the phacoemulsification and side-port incisions, and are used to capture and elevate the pupil margin at 6 and 12 o'clock. Using a slow, steady stretching of the pupil vertically (Figure 6.8) (known as the Luther Frye maneuver), the surgeon stretches the pupillary margin. The hooks are then used to capture and elevate the pupil margin at 3 and 9 o'clock and to stretch the pupil horizontally. Following injection of additional viscoelastic material, this will nearly always result in adequate enlargement of the pupil. Rarely, one will need to augment the stretching with a series of miniature sphincterotomies made with Vannas scissors. Other options are to stretch the pupil with flexible hooks (Grieshaber) placed through the cornea, or to perform a sector iridectomy.

When no red reflex is present, due to the presence of a white cataract or densely brunescent lens, it may be helpful to stain the lens capsule with indocyanine green, which aids in visualizing the capsule during performance of the capsulorhexis. This is done with a 1:10 dilution (with balanced salt solution) of the dye supplied for intravenous use in angiography. One fills the anterior chamber with air and then applies a few drops of the diluted dye to the surface of the lens capsule, using a 30-gauge cannula through the paracentesis. The anterior chamber is then rinsed with balanced salt solution and filled with viscoelastic, prior to making the capsulorhexis.

A continuous tear capsulorhexis (5–7 mm in diameter, depending upon the pupil size) is made with a bent needle cystotome and Utratta forceps. If the view of the leading edge of the capsular tear is obscured by pigment, blood or air bubbles, one may inject more viscoelastic agent to drive the obscuring material to the side. If the iris is in the way, it may be pushed aside with a Kuglen hook or second instrument or nondispersive viscoelastic such as sodium hyaluronate. As one proceeds with the capsulorhexis, visualization of the capsule flap is aided by folding it back upon itself before letting go to regrasp further along the tear. The 'napkin-fold' of the capsule is visible above the surface of the lens as a light reflex, and the slack in the folded capsule helps prevent inadvertent tearing to the periphery of the lens as the capsule is regrasped (technique of Manus Kraff). This technique, allows maximum control during the tear, minimizing the risk of peripheral extension. Cortical cleaving hydrodissection (technique of Howard Fine) is performed with a 27-gauge cannula on a 3-ml syringe filled with balanced salt solution. It is preferable not to perform hydrodissection at the 6 o'clock position, as the cannula would be lying over the center of the lens and would tend to prevent the lens nucleus from rising, thereby retarding the spread of the fluid wave. It is also best not to inject the fluid into the cortex, so as to separate the cortex from the nucleus, but rather to use it to separate, as much as possible, the cortex from the capsule. If the cannula is passed for 2 or 3 mm just under and parallel to the surface of the capsule at 3 or 9 o'clock, the fluid wave will tend to free the cortex as well as the enclosed nucleus from the capsule. When the lens nucleus rises, signaling that the wave of fluid has passed underneath it, the cannula can then be used to push down on the central lens, forcing the fluid wave to come back forward, circumferentially, further separating cortex from capsule. We do not favor performance of hydrodelineation, which is injection of fluid deep into the cortex to separate the cortex from the nucleus, as this results in a loss of visibility through the cortex and, by swelling of the cortex, inhibits subsequent rotation of the lens material within the bag.

The cannula tip is then turned to a vertical orientation and driven 2 mm into the lens material just at the capsulorhexis border in the 1 o'clock position, and pulled counterclockwise toward 11 o'clock, rotating and mobilizing the lens nucleus and cortical material.

PHACOEMULSIFICATION

Despite the introduction and popularity of chopping techniques in cataract surgery, there is still much to be said for the use of a divide and conquer cracking technique of nuclear disassembly (technique of Howard Gimbel), particularly in a case with a shallow anterior chamber, a small pupil, a flaccid iris, and a hard lens.

To ensure visibility of the capsulorhexis edge and of the nucleus, the cortex is first aspirated within the area of the capsulorhexis with the phacoemulsification tip. Then a deep groove is fashioned within the confines of the capsulorhexis. A critical feature of making the groove and later of the intersecting cross-groove, is the use of downslope sculpting. In this technique, a Kelman phacoemulsification tip with a 15° posterior curve (Alcon, Fort Worth, TX) enters the nucleus slightly away from the edge of the capsulorhexis at 12 o'clock and shaves out nuclear material to about one-third of the tip depth with each of several passes. Each pass is alternately shifted slightly to the left or right, so that a groove is made that is 1.5 times as wide as the phacoemulsification tip, wide enough to allow the McCool sleeve on the phacoemulsification tip. It should also be able to enter the groove as it deepens, without pushing the nucleus away from the tip.

The path of the groove is concave, with an initial downslope above, a motion straight across in the center and then an upslope on the far side, stopping short of the capsulorhexis at 6 o'clock. This path parallels the curvature of the posterior capsule, and is a far safer way to make a deep groove than the common technique of beginning the groove near the center of the lens and then doing only upsloping towards 6 o'clock.

Beginner surgeons are often reluctant to do downsloping, in which the phacoemulsification tip is tilted down and thus not as easily seen, for fear that it will penetrate the posterior capsule. With experience, one becomes assured that nuclear sclerotic lenses are quite thick in the central region in which the groove is being created. In addition, the technique has the following advantages: (i) cutting away from the edge of the capsulorhexis superiorly is a more precise and safe way of avoiding cutting the anterior capsule than trying to cut toward it, (ii) downslope sculpting allows one to shave off a uniform amount of nuclear material with each pass, like planing wood, without occluding the phaco-emulsification tip, while upslope sculpting usually results in occlusion of the phacoemulsification tip at the end of a pass under the capsulorhexis edge below, with a resultant build-up of vacuum that suddenly tugs the lens towards the tip, and (iii) downslope sculpting allows one to gradually approach the posterior capsule with strokes that are parallel to it, a much safer way than trying to get deep enough by cutting in a direction somewhat perpendicular to the posterior capsule and then trying to stop just short of it.

After sculpting the initial groove, the nucleus is rotated 90°, using both the phacoemulsification tip and the second instrument (Drysdale spatula introduced through the paracentesis) to turn it, so that there is minimal stress on the zonular diaphragm.

One may then engage the far edge of the groove with the Drysdale spatula (Figure 6.9a) and push the nucleus 1–2 mm toward 6 o'clock, displacing the nucleus within the capsular bag (Figure 6.9b). This allows one to perform downslope sculpting for the cross groove further in the periphery of the nucleus, with the effect that one can create a 7 mm groove through a 5-mm capsulorhexis and 5-mm pupil (Figure 6.9c).

After further rotations and sculpting with nuclear displacement, the nucleus is fractured into quadrants using the phacoemulsification tip and Drysdale spatula. Complete fractures are essential to allow controlled removal of the nuclear quadrants. Each quadrant is then mobilized sequentially in the following fashion: (i) tilting it outward with the phacoemulsification tip so that the posterior

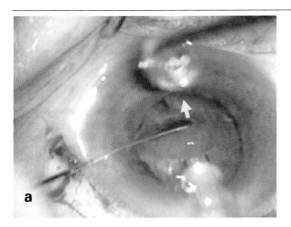

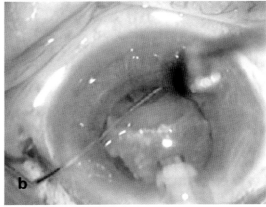

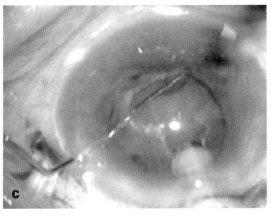

Figure 6.9(a) After formation of a groove in the lens nucleus, and a 90° rotation of the lens, the inferior edge of the groove is engaged by the Drysdale spatula. The nucleus will be pushed inferiorly in the direction of the arrow. (b) The nucleus has been pushed inferiorly with a Drysdale spatula, bringing some of the superior nucleus out from under the anterior capsule and into position for downslope sculpting with the phacoemulsification tip. (c) After several strokes of downslope sculpting, a cross-groove is partially formed.

portion lifts up slightly from the posterior capsule, allowing the Drysdale spatula to pass under the quadrant, (ii) lifting it from beneath with the spatula and rotating it into a horizontal orientation, and (iii) phacoemulsifying it in the center of the capsular bag, away from the corneal endothelium and the edge of the capsulorhexis. After a quadrant is removed, the remaining quadrants are pushed around counterclockwise in the capsular bag, so that the remaining quadrants keep the capsular bag expanded on the right side of the piece being emulsified, while the Drysdale spatula protects the posterior capsule on the left side or directly underneath the quadrant.

CORTICAL ASPIRATION

When cortical cleaving hydrodissection has been achieved, and the nucleus removed, the anterior cortex will hang free from the anterior capsule. The free edge of the anterior cortex is then easily engaged in the cortical aspiration tip, with little risk of engaging the capsule, and little force is required to pull the cortex free from the capsule, thus minimizing stress on the capsule and zonular fibers. Angled aspiration tips are particularly helpful for removing subincisional cortex (Rhein Medical, Tampa, FL). It is highly preferable when engaging and pulling cortex free from the capsular bag to *always keep the aspiration port pointing up*, and to pivot the handpiece from side to side to reach the cortex, and not to rotate the port to one side or the other, which increases the risk of engaging and pulling on the more fragile posterior capsule. When it is difficult to maintain a well-inflated capsular bag, the surgeon can place a temporary stitch to narrow the incision which will help reduce leakage from the wound. While the viscoelastic is still present, the surgeon can create a paracentesis 180° away from the phacoemulsification incision, and pass a 27-guage cannula across the anterior chamber to aspirate the cortex. Alternatively, one may remove subincisional cortex with the irrigation/aspiration tip once the intraocular lens is placed, since the lens will hold the posterior capsule away from the aspiration port.

INTRAOCULAR LENS INSERTION

After filling the capsular bag and anterior chamber with a viscoelastic agent, a foldable intraocular lens can be inserted with either a lens inserter or forceps. Either an acrylic or silicone lens can be easily inserted through a small pupil with little risk of damage to the posterior capsule.

MITOMYCIN C APPLICATION

After removal of the viscoelastic agent and injection of acetylcholine (Miochol, Ciba Vision, Atlanta, GA) into the anterior chamber to constrict the pupil, the surgeon places a temporary 10-0 nylon suture in the phacoemulsification wound to obtain watertight closure. Two thin pieces are cut from the sides of a cellulose spear sponge and are placed on any disposable plastic surface. Mitomycin C (Mutamycin, Bristol-Myers, Evansville, IN) 0.4–0.5 mg/ml is applied to the sponges with a tuberculin syringe, causing them to swell to about $6 \times 4 \times 1$ mm (Figure 6.10). Westcott scissors are used to create a subconjunctival pocket in the superior temporal and superior nasal quadrants. The sponges are then placed to each side of the superior rectus insertion using nontoothed forceps, and arranged so that they touch each other anteriorly over the phacoemulsification wound. The conjunctival flap is then pulled forward with nontoothed forceps (to avoid puncturing the conjunctiva), with one tine above and one tine below the flap (so as not to tear the flap), and the flap left in place over the sponges for 5 minutes. The sponges are then removed and copious irrigation is performed with saline (Figure 6.11). (The technique of using thin sponges over a wide area under a fornix flap has been shown by Peng Khaw to produce broader blebs that are not excessively ischemic or thin, and have little tendency to leak or become infected. We previously used one 5 $\times$ 4 mm thick sponge, which was used for the cases reported in Tables 6.1 and 6.2, but also resulted in blebs that were smaller and more ischemic.)

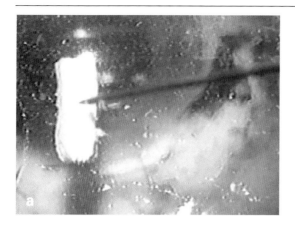 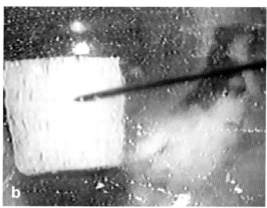

Figure 6.10(a) A piece cut from the edge of a cellulose spear sponge is about to be hydrated with mitomycin C. The solution will be applied with a Tuberculin syringe through a 30-gauge needle. (b) The same piece of sponge has now been hydrated, and swells to $5 \times 5 \times 1$ mm.

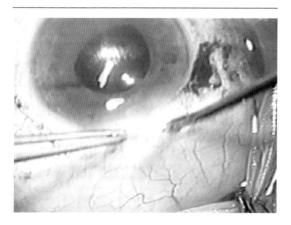

Figure 6.11 After application of the mitomycin C sponge for 5 minutes, the sponge was carefully removed and placed in a special bag for transporting antimetabolites (not shown). Now the scleral surface and underside of the conjunctival–Tenon's flap are being irrigated with saline using a 20-ml syringe and a cannula.

CONSTRUCTION OF THE 'SAFETY VALVE' INCISION

A Kelly Descemet's punch (0.75 mm, Storz, St Louis, MO) is advanced (horizontal to the surface) into the tunnel incision, the posterior lip of the wound is engaged, and the punch is rotated to a vertical orientation. The barrel of the punch is then gently pushed forward towards the center of the cornea and a bite of the posterior lip of the wound is punched out and removed.

Counterintuitively, the surgeon's pushing the barrel of the punch towards the center of the cornea while punching aids in cutting the posterior lip. Pulling the barrel of the punch towards the surgeon compresses the tissue of the posterior lip and results in cutting a furrow that is not full-thickness. If that furrow extends to the external tunnel mouth, it will be difficult to avoid overfiltration. After taking about two or three punches in a radial line in the posterior lip, the surgeon will have created a canal that stops about 0.5–1 mm short of the external phacoemulsification tunnel opening (Figure 6.12). This wound construction creates a valve-like structure.

A peripheral iridectomy is then performed by the surgeon by passing 0.12 forceps along the phacoemulsification tunnel, dipping the tines to grasp peripheral iris, pulling the iris to the tunnel mouth (Figure 6.13), and cutting the iris with Vannas scissors. The iris is reposited by gently stroking the wound with a 30-gauge cannula, starting posteriorly and going anteriorly. The pupil should become round and the peripheral iridectomy should be visible through the peripheral cornea. The tunnel mouth is then held open with a 0.12 forceps to inspect the tunnel for any residual iris pigment,

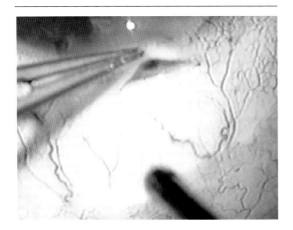

Figure 6.12 The mouth of the tunnel incision is lifted to reveal the canal within the base of the tunnel created by taking two or three punches with a Kelly Descemet's punch (0.75 mm, Storz, St Louis, MO). After allowing the tunnel to close, balanced salt solution will be placed into the anterior chamber to test the intraocular pressure. A pressure of 4–6 mmHg is desirable prior to placing sutures.

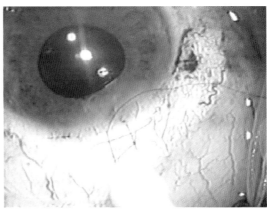

Figure 6.14 After tying two 10-0 nylon sutures loosely in the scleral tunnel mouth, and re-forming the anterior chamber with balanced salt solution through the paracentesis, a cellulose spear sponge is used to absorb effluent at the tunnel mouth, allowing one to judge when equilibrium flow is reached.

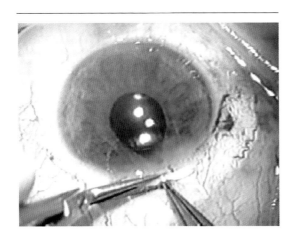

Figure 6.13 The 0.12 forceps are passed into the tunnel incision, dipped to grasp the iris 1 mm away from the iris insertion, and bring the iris to the mouth of the wound, where angled Vannas scissors will be used to perform a small iridectomy.

which if present can be wiped away with a cellulose spear sponge.

The valve function of the 'safety valve incision' is then tested. Balanced salt solution is injected into the anterior chamber with a 30-gauge cannula through the paracentesis until the pressure is high enough to start flow through the tunnel. The flow is then estimated with a spear sponge which absorbs fluid from the mouth of the tunnel (Figure 6.14). The IOP at equilibrium flow can then be estimated by depressing the center of the cornea with a 30-gauge needle on a tuberculin syringe. The goal is to have the pressure be about 4–6 mmHg prior to the placement of any sutures. If the resistance is too great, additional punching of the posterior lip of the internal entry may be performed. Two sutures are then placed to close the wound. The goal is for the IOP to be approximately 8–12 mmHg, which is estimated by pushing down on the center of the cornea with a 30-gauge cannula (Figure 6.15). This strategy can be highly successful in setting the eye pressure in its target range. If the IOP increases postoperatively due to healing of the conjunctiva–Tenon's capsule layers, laser suture lysis of one or both of the scleral tunnel sutures can help decrease the IOP. The 'safety valve incision' prevents IOPs from going lower than approximately 5 mmHg which provides some safety against severe hypotony. In addition, if suprachoroidal hemorrhage occurs, the valve-like incision closes which causes the IOP to increase and to halt the bleeding.

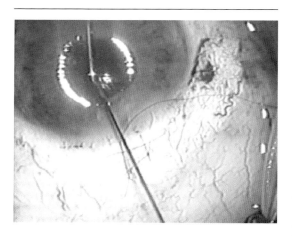

Figure 6.15 The IOP is estimated by pushing down on the center of the cornea with the bend of a 30-gauge cannula. A fairly standard estimate is achieved by pushing down just enough to create a circle of reflected light from the microscope measuring approximately 3 mm in diameter.

CONJUNCTIVAL FLAP CLOSURE

The conjunctiva is closed with a series of three mattress sutures. The first suture is a central mattress which anchors the conjunctival flap at 12 o'clock (Figure 6.16a). A 10-0 nylon suture is anchored in to the sclera 1 mm posterior to and parallel to the peripheral cornea. The needle is passed through equal bites of Tenon's capsule and conjunctiva and then back down through them. The knot is tied underneath the conjunctival flap. Pursestring mattress sutures are then used to pull the conjunctiva–Tenon's taut over the limbus and to close the relaxing incisions in the conjunctiva. The needle is passed through sclera at the temporal limbus, and the conjunctiva–Tenon's is pulled downwards and outwards to be impaled upon the tip of the needle as it emerges from the sclera. The needle is passed up through the conjunctiva–Tenon's flap, turned around and then a series of bites is taken to close the relaxing incision in a pursestring closure. This and a similar suture placed nasally produce watertight closure along the limbus. The anterior chamber is then filled with balanced saline so that the fluid will pass through the filtration site and fill the bleb (Figure 16.6b). If the bleb holds fluid without a leak along the limbus, the closure is adequate. If not, additional mattress sutures are placed to tighten the closure along the limbus.

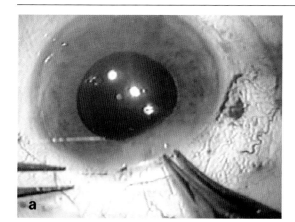
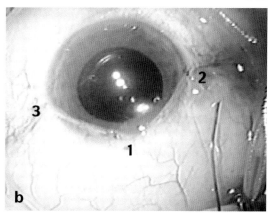

Figure 6.16(a) An anchoring stitch of 10-0 nylon is passed at half-thickness through limbal sclera, in front of the filtration site. It is then passed vertically up through equal bites of Tenon's capsule and conjunctiva about 0.5 mm from the limbus, and then back down through. The knot is tied underneath the conjunctival flap. (b) After placement of the anchoring stitch at 12 o'clock (location 1), pursestring mattress sutures are placed at 9 o'clock (location 2) and at 3 o'clock (location 3) to anchor the conjunctival flap to sclera and to close the relaxing incisions. Balanced salt solution is then instilled into the anterior chamber through the paracentesis. The bleb should inflate. Fluoroscein can be used to check for leak along the limbal closure. Additional buried mattress sutures may be needed along the limbal closure to obtain watertight closure, if there is a leak.

CONCLUSIONS

One-site combined phacoemulsification and tra-beculectomy with mitomycin C is an excellent approach for patients with cataract and glaucoma. Equal IOP control and visual field stability were achieved with either phacoemulsification or extra-capsular cataract surgery in our clinical trial. Thus, we conclude that one need not do a two-site combined procedure, nor use phacoemulsification, to achieve optimal glaucoma control after cataract extraction.

FURTHER READING

AGIS Investigators. The Advanced Glaucoma Intervention Study (AGIS): 7. The relationship between control of intraocular pressure and visual field deterioration. Am J Ophthalmol 2000; 130: 429–40.

Fine IH, Packer M, Hoffman RS. Prevention of posterior segment complications of phacoemulsification. Ophthalmol Clin North Am 2001; 14: 581–93.

Gimbel HV. Nucleofractis phacoemulsification through a small pupil. Can J Ophthalmol 1992; 27: 115.

Jampel HD, Friedman DS, Lubomski LH et al. Effect of technique on intraocular pressure after combined cataract and glaucoma surgery. Ophthalmology 2002; 109: 2215–2224.

Joos KM, Bueche MJ, Palmberg PF, Feuer WJ, Grajewski AL. One year followup results of combined mitomycin C trabeculectomy and extracapsular cataract extraction. Ophthalmology 1994; 102: 76–83.

Kraff MC. Lecture given at the Current Concepts in Ophthalmology Meeting, (San Diego Eye Bank), in LaJolla, CA, June, 1990.

Khaw P. Technique of using antimetabolites. In: Alm A, ed. The Gullstrand Foundation Meeting, April 1, 2001. CD-ROM. Uppsala University, Uppsala, Sweden.

Palmberg P. Combined cataract and glaucoma surgery with mitomycin. Ophthalmol Clin North Am 1995; 8: 365–81.

Palmberg P. Risk factors for glaucoma progression: Where does intraocular pressure fit in? [Editorial]. Arch Ophthalmol 2001; 119: 897–8.

Palmberg P. Target pressure. In: Alm A, ed, The Gullstrand Foundation Meeting, April 1, 2001. CD-ROM. Uppsala University, Uppsala, Sweden.

Palmberg P. How clinical trial results are changing our thinking about target pressures. Curr Opin Ophthalmol 2002; 13: 85–8.

Suner IJ, Greenfield DS, Miller MP, Nicolela MT, Palmberg PF. Hypotony maculopathy following filtering surgery with Mitomycin C: Incidence and treatment. Ophthalmology 1997; 104: 207–14.

7. Two-site combined cataract extraction and trabeculectomy

Joseph Caprioli and Michelle Banks

INDICATIONS

When carefully considered, the combination of cataract extraction with trabeculectomy is a valuable surgical option in the management of patients with coexisting glaucoma and cataract. Important variables to consider when deciding whether to perform simultaneous or sequential cataract extraction and trabeculectomy include the level of intraocular pressure (IOP) control and the degree of optic nerve damage. Optic nerve damage can be categorized clinically according to the amount of visual field loss. A simple method of interpretation would suggest that early nerve damage is associated with little or no visual field damage, moderate damage shows field defects in one hemifield and advanced damage results in visual field loss in both hemifields.

As depicted in Figure 7.1, an algorithm may aid the surgeon in choosing the appropriate surgical approach in patients with both glaucoma and cataract. The surgical approach can follow one of three sequences that either separate or combine the two procedures. Simultaneous cataract extraction

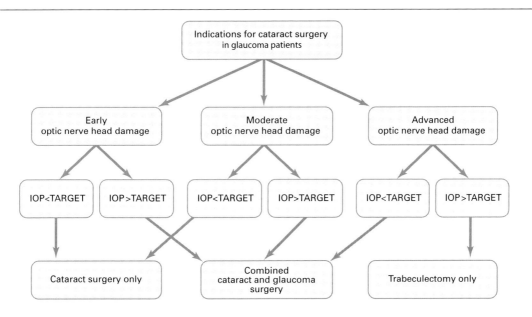

Figure 7.1 Algorithm for the surgical approach to patients with coexisting glaucoma and cataracts.

The clinician must first determine the severity of optic nerve damage based on the amount of visual field loss. Patients with early damage have little or no visual field changes, while patients with moderate damage have a glaucomatous visual change in only one hemifield. Severe optic nerve damage is characterized by visual field loss in both hemifields. The target intraocular pressure (IOP) is determined by the clinician. (Courtesy of Caprioli J. Combined phacoemulsification and trabeculectomy. In: Albert D (ed) Ophthalmic Surgery: Principles and Techniques. 1999, Cambridge, MA: Blackwell Science, Inc. Reproduced with permission from Blackwell Publishers Inc.)

and trabeculectomy is recommended for patients with either inadequately controlled IOP and early to moderate optic nerve damage, or in patients with severe nerve damage with adequately controlled IOP. Cataract surgery alone is sufficient for patients with well-controlled IOP and early or moderate optic nerve damage. Trabeculectomy alone is most appropriate if the IOP is not controlled in the presence of severe or advancing optic nerve damage.

Many factors contribute to the success or failure of surgical procedures. Recent advances in the surgical management of cataracts and glaucoma, including temporal clear cornea approach for phacoemulsification and antimetabolite use in filtration surgery, have improved surgical outcomes in patients with coexistent cataract and glaucoma. With the evolution of extracapsular cataract extraction (ECCE) from intracapsular cataract extraction, there has been a growing interest in combining cataract extraction with trabeculectomy. However, before the development of small incision surgery, the results of combined trabeculectomy and ECCE were less than favorable. When compared with trabeculectomy alone, the combination of trabeculectomy and cataract extraction did not provide an equivalent reduction in IOP. ECCE is likely associated with more postoperative inflammation when compared with small incision phacoemulsification. The increased inflammation following ECCE generally lengthens the recovery period and has been found to contribute to trabeculectomy failure. In addition, the ECCE technique involves manipulation of the conjunctiva which can also negatively influence the outcome of filtration surgery. Because of the less than optimal results, the combination of large incision ECCE and trabeculectomy was not widely adopted for many patients with glaucoma and cataracts.

In the past decade, numerous developments have advanced the success of both cataract and glaucoma surgery. In contrast with ECCE, the temporal clear cornea incision for cataract extraction avoids manipulation of the conjunctiva and preserves healthy tissue essential for the success of the filtering bleb. The use of intraoperative antimetabolites is more likely to result in satisfactory reduction of IOP in patients with combined glaucoma and cataract.

The combination of small incision phacoemulsification and trabeculectomy can be performed through a common incision or separate incisions. The two-site technique of cataract extraction combined with trabeculectomy is the approach that we have studied and favor, and this will be discussed here.

SURGICAL PROCEDURE

The list of instruments required is given in Box 7.1.

Box 7.1 Surgical instruments

Jaffe lid speculum
No. 75 Beaver blade
3.0-mm diamond keratome blade
27-gauge cannula
30-gauge cannula
Cystotome
Utrata capsulorhexis forceps
10-0 nylon suture
4-0 silk suture
French (tissue) forceps
Westcott scissors, blunt
No. 67 Beaver blade
18-gauge wet-field cautery
Weck-cell sponges
Cotton-tip applicators
Vannas scissors
Colibri forceps, 0.12 mm
De Wecker scissors
Collagen shield
Sterile eye pad
Fox shield
Balanced salt solution irrigator
Viscoelastic agent
Barraquer iris spatula
Sinskey intraocular lens manipulating hook
Muscle hook
Large tooth superior rectus fixation forceps
Tying forceps, angled
Tying forceps, straight
Mosquito forceps
Needle holder, standard
Needle holder, micro

CATARACT EXTRACTION

DILATION

Preoperatively, two sets of topical mydriatic agents, preferably, tropicamide (1%, Mydriacyl) and phenylephrine (2.5%) are instilled approximately 20–30 minutes prior to surgery. Despite heroic attempts at pharmacologic dilation, patients treated with long-term miotics may have irreversibly miotic pupils or posterior synechiae that require intraoperative manipulation.

ANESTHESIA

In spite of an increasing trend toward the use of topical anesthesia during phacoemulsification, retrobulbar anesthesia is preferable for combined cataract extraction and trabeculectomy. Intravenous midazolam (0.5 mg, Versed) and/or propofol (50 mg, Diprivan) may be administered to the patient for sedation, although the final choice should be left to the anesthesiologist. A retrobulbar injection, usually lidocaine (1%), provides the patient with effective anesthesia. This level of anesthesia is especially important for patient comfort during procedures that may require iris manipulation or extensive dissection of the conjunctiva. The retrobulbar anesthetic is supplemented with a 1.0 ml injection of lidocaine given above the superior rectus muscle which provides comfort during placement of the superior rectus bridle suture at the beginning of the trabeculectomy and during closure of the conjunctiva. Alternatively, a traction suture placed in the superior cornea can provide excellent exposure and minimize potential scarring and hemorrhage in the filtering site.

INCISION

A clear corneal incision eliminates conjunctival manipulation prior to performing the trabeculectomy. The surgeon may opt to perform clear corneal cataract extraction through an incision located either temporally or superiorly. We prefer the temporal approach (Figure 7.2). For the temporal clear corneal approach, the surgeon sits at the temporal side of the patient. To begin the procedure, a paracentesis track is created through clear

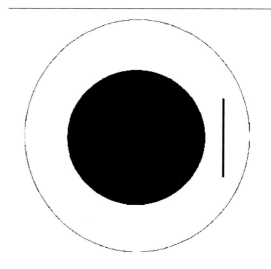

Figure 7.2 Clear cornea incision for phacoemulsification.

The surgeon is seated temporally. The incision is made at the temporal or 3 o'clock position. Note the widely dilated pupil which facilitates subsequent capsulorhexis and phacoemulsification.

cornea with a No. 75 Beaver blade approximately 2 clock hours or 60° clockwise or counterclockwise from the anticipated cataract wound. A small incision is preferred for cataract extraction. At the surgeon's 12 o'clock position, a temporal clear corneal incision is made with a 3.2-mm diamond keratome. A moist cotton swab is used to stabilize the globe while making the incision to minimize trauma to the conjunctiva. The globe can also be stabilized by grasping the edge of the paracentesis with a 0.12 forceps. Following capsulorhexis, adequate hydrodissection of the nucleus and epinucleus as described in Chapters 2 and 6 is essential. This allows free manipulation of the nucleus during phacoemulsification and minimizes the chance of lens capsule or zonule rupture.

PHACOEMULSIFICATION

Standard phacoemulsification is performed through the temporal clear corneal incision. The phacoemulsification machine, settings and technique depend on the individual surgeon's preference. Initially, we prefer moderate phacoemulsification power and aspiration flow rate with low vacuum settings. Phacoemulsification on patients with glaucoma and especially those patients with coexisting pseudoex-foliation requires special consideration since these patients are at increased risk for zonular dehiscence and lens subluxation. Attention to the movement of the lens is important during phacoemulsification. To avoid frank zonular dehiscence and lens subluxation, phacoemulsification should be performed gently in an effort to not overly manipulate the lens. Nucleus sculpting can be safely performed with low vacuum, low aspiration flow rate, low infusion and increased power if necessary. Another important obstacle during phacoemulsification is persistent miosis which is often found in patients who have a history of long-term miotic use or posterior synechiae, as well as pseudoexfoliation. Pupils less than 4 mm in diameter after dilation should be enlarged with viscoelastic following nasal and temporal sphincterotomies. In the presence of posterior synechiae, a blunt sweep, such as a Barraquer spatula, can be used to lyse the adhesions prior to performing the sphincterotomies.

LENS INSERTION
Foldable intraocular lenses have facilitated advancements in small incision cataract extraction. A foldable silicone plate haptic or single piece acrylic intraocular lens can be inserted into the capsular bag using a lens inserter or injector through the clear cornea incision. For cases when sulcus fixation is required, a three piece foldable IOL should be used.

WOUND CLOSURE
The small clear corneal incision must be closed securely with a suture. A single 10-0 nylon suture is placed half-thickness to approximate the edges of the temporal clear cornea incision. The knot is buried into the corneal stroma. At the completion of the cataract extraction, intracameral carbachol is injected to constrict the pupil and aid subsequence creation of the peripheral iridectomy. Additional balanced salt solution (BSS) is injected through the paracentesis port in order to firm the globe. The wound is checked for leakage with gentle pressure with a Weck cell sponge. A tight seal at the temporal clear corneal incision reduces the incidence of

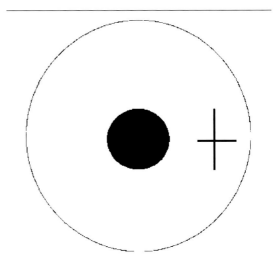

Figure 7.3 Completion of temporal clear cornea phacoemulsification. Following nucleus and cortical removal, a foldable intraocular lens is inserted into the capsular bag. At the completion of the phacoemulsification, the corneal wound is closed using 10-0 nylon suture. Note the constricted pupil following injection of intracameral carbachol. The anterior chamber is re-pressurized with balanced salt solution.

leakage and facilitates dissection of the scleral flap during the trabeculectomy (Figure 7.3).

TRABECULECTOMY

POSITION
The trabeculectomy is performed superiorly. Therefore, after cataract extraction the surgeon should change position to the superior side, or head, of the patient, with the assistant seated temporally.

FORNIX- VERSUS LIMBUS-BASED-FLAPS
The conjunctival flap may be either fornix-based or limbus-based. A fornix-based conjunctival flap generally provides better exposure, but may result in less protection against postoperative leaks. For the fornix-based flap, a 6-0 silk is placed through mid-stroma of the cornea just anterior to the limbus and used for downward traction of the globe. Using French forceps and Westcott scissors, a peritomy is performed at the superior limbus from the

10 to 2 o'clock position. After completion of the standard trabeculectomy, which is described in Chapters 3 and 6, the conjunctiva is closed tightly with interrupted 9-0 vicryl sutures at the nasal and temporal most edges of the wound. The limbal sutures should include a small bite of limbal sclera along with conjunctiva. This promotes a tight seal at the limbus and will help to reduce the incidence of significant leaks.

When using antimetabolites in a combined cataract and glaucoma procedure, a secure, water-tight wound is critical, and is best assured with a standard limbus-based conjunctival flap. For the limbus-based approach, a 4-0 silk suture is passed beneath the insertion of the superior rectus muscle and clamped to the drape superiorly to provide downward traction of the eye and good exposure of the superior limbus. A clear corneal traction stitch described above can be used instead and may interfere less with conjunctival closure. Tissue forceps, such as French forceps and blunt Westcott scissors are used to incise the conjunctiva and Tenon's capsule just over the anterior edge of the superior rectus insertion. Care is taken to avoid the superior rectus muscle insertion and overlying vessels. The episclera is incised anterior to the muscle insertion. Dissection along bare sclera is continued anteriorly to the limbus. At the limbus, a 4 × 4 mm square scleral flap is outlined with cautery while the assistant gently elevates the conjunctival flap with smooth forceps by grasping Tenon's layer only. The scleral flap can be triangular, square, rectangular, or trapezoidal.

USE OF ANTIMETABOLITES

Mitomycin-C (MMC) is our antimetabolite of choice for intraoperative application. A thin piece of Weck cell sponge soaked in the desired concentration (usually 0.2 mg/ml) of MMC is placed on the scleral bed. Conjunctiva and Tenon's are repositioned over the MMC sponge for a desired amount of time (usually 1 minute). Alternative MMC concentrations and/or durations of application should be considered in patients with preexisting conjunctival scarring or risk factors for trabeculectomy failure, including previous failed trabeculectomy.

Following MMC application, BSS is then used to copiously irrigate the area.

SCLERAL FLAP AND KERATO-SCLEROSTOMY

Dissection of a half-thickness scleral flap is performed with a No. 67 Beaver blade and should be extended anteriorly into the clear cornea. The assistant releases the Tenon's capsule and grasps the scleral flap with the tissue forceps. A 3 mm sclerostomy is formed with the No. 75 Beaver blade guided radial to the base of the flap and Vannas scissors circumferentially just posteriorly then anteriorly (Figure 7.4). A basal iridectomy is performed with DeWecker scissors. Prolapsed iris is repositioned and the scleral flap is reapproximated at an appropriate tension using two interrupted 10-0 nylon sutures at the apices of the flap. Target postoperative IOP, the preoperative rate of glaucomatous progression, and the risk of shallow anterior chamber and/or hypotony are factors which influence the appropriate tension of the scleral sutures.

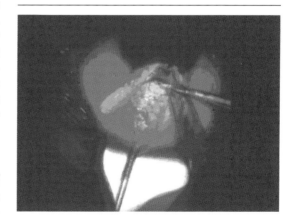

Figure 7.4 Sclerostomy performed with Vannas scissors.

The superior rectus bridle suture is shown rotating the globe inferiorly. The scleral flap is retracted anteriorly by the assistant using tissue forceps. A No. 75 blade has been used to enter the anterior chamber radial to the base of the scleral flap in two areas approximately 3 mm apart. Vannas scissors are shown performing the sclerostomy by guiding the scissors circumferentially to the base of the scleral flap at the anterior edge of the radial incision and then posteriorly to free a rectangular piece of sclera.

WOUND CLOSURE

The conjunctiva–Tenon's wound is closed with a single running 9-0 Vicryl suture. The surgeon should gently grasp the edge of Tenon's capsule with tissue forceps while the conjunctival edge is identified and elevated with the needle tip of the 9-0 Vicryl suture. Taking a small bite, the needle is passed near the anterior edge of the conjunctiva and then through the free edge of Tenon's capsule on the same side. On the opposite side, a larger bite is taken as the needle is passed through the Tenon's capsule first and then the conjunctiva. Care should be taken to include both layers of Tenon's capsule and conjunctiva with each bite in order to ensure watertight closure (Figure 7.5).

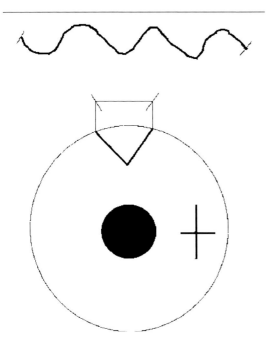

Figure 7.5 Completion of separate incision phacoemulsification and trabeculectomy.

Temporal clear cornea approach to phacoemulsification minimizes conjunctival manipulation. A single 10-0 nylon suture secures the wound. The trabeculectomy is performed at the 12 o'clock position with the formation of a diffuse bleb superiorly. The conjunctiva–Tenon's wound is closed with a running 9-0 Vicryl suture. (Courtesy of Ali BH and Caprioli J. Cataract surgery in the presence of a filtering bleb. Operative Techniques in Cataract and Refractive Surgery, Vol 2, No 2 (June), 1999; 58–64.)

HAZARDS

MIOTIC PUPILS

Long-term use of topical miotics may cause inelastic, miotic pupils. In addition, patients may have posterior synechiae that inhibit adequate pupil dilation. Because adequate pupil dilation simplifies cataract extraction, special procedures may have to be performed during cataract extraction in glaucoma patients with miotic pupils. Small sphincterotomies at the nasal and temporal aspects of the pupil can aid in enlarging the pupil diameter (Figure 7.6). This is in contrast to the technique in which the entire fibrotic pupil is stretched which causes multiple sphincter tears and tends to increase postoperative inflammation. Iris hooks, though time consuming, can be placed to maintain an adequate diameter in the setting of a small pupil. Iris manipulators can be used to stretch the pupil and create small tears in the sphincter, thereby, increasing pupil diameter. We prefer to lyse adhesions with a blunt instrument such as a Barraquer spatula. Once adhesions have been lysed and small temporal and nasal sphincterectomies have been performed, viscoelastic injection usually provides a sufficiently dilated pupil through which phacoemulsification can be performed safely.

IRIS PROLAPSE

The use of long-term miotics in patients with glaucoma can cause atrophy of the iris. An atrophic iris has a tendency to prolapse through the corneal wound during cataract extraction. Avoiding a peripherally placed wound near the iris base and performing proper wound construction can help prevent iris prolapse. Placement of a cohesive type viscoelastic material (e.g. Viscoat) at the base of the iris can aid in management of iris prolapse through the wound.

BLEEDING

Prolonged use of topical antiglaucoma medications, particularly epinephrine and pilocarpine, increases the risk of intraoperative bleeding. Because intraoperative bleeding is associated with an increased risk of trabeculectomy failure, hemo-

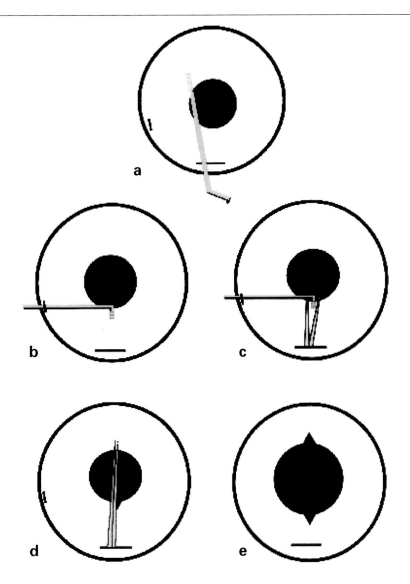

Figure 7.6 Sphincterotomies for miotic pupils.

The miotic pupil may be enlarged surgically. (a) Adhesions between the iris and lens are lysed using a blunt instrument inserted through the temporal incision. (b) A clear cornea counter incision is made through which the remaining adhesions are lysed. (c, d) Nasal and temporal sphincterectomies are performed. A viscoelastic material is injected into the anterior chamber to enlarge the pupil. (Courtesy of Caprioli J. Combined phacoemulsification and trabeculectomy. Ophthalmic Surgery: Principles and Techniques. Cambridge, MA: Blackwell Science, Inc.)

stasis is important. In addition, epinephrine and pilocarpine should be discontinued and replaced with an alternative medication 3–4 weeks prior to surgery whenever feasible.

ZONULAR INSTABILITY

Preoperative recognition of zonular instability can help to avoid intraoperative complications such as frank dehiscence and vitreous loss. The presence of pseudoexfoliation is an important finding that signals possible zonular instability. In the event that there is no frank zonular dehiscence, careful and gentle phacoemulsification can be performed successfully. We have found two maneuvers particularly useful in performing phacoemulsification in the presence of zonular instability. The first is to perform a large capsulotomy, which aids manipulation of the nucleus and decreases traction on the zonule throughout the procedure. Second, increased phacoemulsification power prevents rocking movement of the lens, which additionally reduces traction on the zonules.

CYSTOID MACULAR EDEMA

Certain antiglaucoma medications, especially epinephrine and prostaglandin analogs, have been associated with the development of cystoid macular edema following cataract extraction and should be avoided postoperatively for 1 month.

CONCLUSION

The management of coexistent cataract and glaucoma can be challenging for the ocular surgeon. Many approaches exist. The best approach is dictated by the amount of optic nerve damage and level of IOP control. Patients with stable glaucoma or less severe optic nerve damage in the presence of cataract may benefit from combined trabeculectomy and cataract extraction. However, patients with severe or progressive optic nerve damage should first undergo trabeculectomy followed by cataract extraction 3–6 months later, if required. With the advent of clear corneal phacoemulsification for cataract extraction and the use of antimetabolites in glaucoma surgery, the outcomes of combined procedures have improved. The two-site combined trabeculectomy and cataract extraction has many theoretical advantages, particularly less conjunctival manipulation, and has become increasingly accepted in the current practice of glaucoma specialists.

FURTHER READING

Ali BH, Caprioli J. Cataract surgery in the presence of a filtering bleb. Operative Techniques in Cataract and Refractive Surgery, 1999; 2: 58–64.

Gaddie IB, Bennet DW. Cystoid macular edema associated with the use of Latanoprost. J Am Optom Assoc 1998; 69: 122–8.

Lyle WA, Jin JC. Comparison of a 3–6-mm incision in combined phacoemulsification trabeculectomy. Am J Ophthalmol 1991; 111: 189–96.

Park HJ, Kwon YH, Weitzman M et al. Temporal corneal phacoemulsification in patients with filtered glaucoma. Arch Ophthalmol 1997; 115: 1375–80.

Simmons ST, Litoff D, Nichols DA, Sherwood MD, Spaeth GL. Extracapsular cataract extraction and posterior chamber intraocular lens implantation combined with trabeculectomy in patients with glaucoma. Am J Ophthalmol 1987; 104: 465–70.

Weitzman M, Caprioli J. Temporal corneal phacoemulsification combined with separate-incision superior trabeculectomy. Ophthal Surg 1995; 26: 271–3.

Williamson TH, Bacon AS, Flanagan DW, Jakeman CM, Jordan K. Combined extracapsular cataract extraction trabeculectomy using a separated corneal incision. Eye 1989; 3: 547–52.

8. Combined cataract and drainage device procedures

Sheila P. Sanders and Richard P. Mills

INTRODUCTION

Glaucoma drainage devices (GDDs) are generally reserved for advanced or complicated cases where a previous trabeculectomy has failed, or cannot be performed due to severe conjunctival changes. GDDs do not usually achieve an intraocular pressure (IOP) as low as trabeculectomy, and are more likely to require postoperative supplemental medications. Visually significant cataracts often coexist in patients with challenging forms of glaucoma. One typical situation occurs following a failed primary trabeculectomy in a phakic eye. The initial glaucoma surgery often induces accelerated cataract progression, and the IOP rises due to bleb failure. The condition of a failed bleb with unacceptable IOP and a visually significant cataract is even more likely if there is an underlying inflammatory or ischemic process. To best provide glaucoma control and visual rehabilitation quickly, a combined GDD and cataract extraction can be performed.

It is unclear whether there is a higher risk of GDD failure if cataract removal is performed at the same time as GDD surgery, rather than as a separate procedure. The risks of immediate postoperative complications, especially inflammation and hypotony, are higher with a combined procedure. However, if a cataract already exists in an eye requiring GDD, it is likely that the cataract will progress more quickly following the glaucoma surgery if it is not removed simultaneously. Sudden failure of IOP control following a second surgery, such as a later cataract extraction, does occur, and is likely due to inflammation and fluctuations in IOP which thicken the GDD bleb wall.

A combined procedure is especially useful in monocular patients seeking rapid visual rehabilitation, or in situations when two separate trips to the operating room are contraindicated by the patient's health or personal circumstances. There is a relative financial benefit to the patient who has a combined procedure. Because of the high risk and considerable effort on the part of both surgeon and patient, a combined cataract and GDD procedure should be offered only when there is reasonable hope for improved vision. Cyclophotocoagulation without lens extraction may be a better choice if the visual potential is extremely poor.

THE SURGICAL APPROACH

SURGICAL PROCEDURES

In general, it is easier to sew the external device to the eye while it is firm, before any entry into the globe is made. It is also easier to perform phacoemulsification prior to insertion of the drainage tube into the eye. Box 8.1 gives the list of instruments required.

Surgeons who are more comfortable with clear corneal cataract surgery may prefer two-site surgery, since the cataract portion will be identical to their usual phacoemulsifcation procedure. A limbal peritomy with fornix-based flap is the ideal approach to any GDD procedure unless there is substantial perilimbal conjunctival scarring. A limbal-based flap places the suture line closer to the device, with a higher risk of wound complications.

Antimetabolites have been used successfully in conjunction with GDDs. However, the success rate is not significantly higher than in non-antimetabolite cases, and may carry some additional risk of increased postoperative complications. There are no specific indications for the use of antimetabolites with GDDs, and they are not recommended for routine cases.

Box 8.1 List of Surgical Instruments

Drugs for retrobulbar block (e.g. lidocaine 1%, bupivicaine 0.75%, wydase) – if general anesthesia is not to be used

Lid speculum

Sauer forceps/large needle driver for rectus traction suture versus smaller needle driver for corneal traction suture

Westcott scissors

Notched straight or Colibri forceps

Cautery – recommend Mentor bipolar 23-gauge tapered blunt tip or bipolar forceps

No. 75 blade or small diamond paracentesis blade

Viscoelastic

23-gauge needle

Titanium needle driver

Stevens scissors

Tying forceps

Suture material : 8-0 Vicryl for conjunctiva, 9-0 nylon or 6.0 Mersilene for device, 5-0 nylon and 7-0 polyglactin for temporary tube ligature, 5-0–7-0 silk for traction suture

Scleral patch material – donor sclera, pericardial tissue, dura mater, or fascia lata

Glaucoma drainage device – Ahmed, Molteno, Baerveldt, or Krupin

Diamond or metal keratome

Cystotome and/or Utrata forceps

BSS syringe/27-gauge cannula

Phacoemulsification handpiece

Chopper/cracking instrument (Siebel, Drysdale, Lester, etc.)

Sinskey hook

Irrigation/aspiration handpiece (single or bimanual)

Anterior vitrectomy unit on standby

Lens insertion/folding instruments

Drugs for injection (e.g. solumedrol, tobramycin)

Optional – indocyanine green dye, iris hooks, nonpreserved lidocaine

Intraocular lens implant

Patients who are at high risk for hypotony, such as younger, high myopes, could undergo a two-stage shunt procedure. The device is sewn to the external eye during an initial surgery, and is introduced into the anterior chamber during a subsequent procedure after the fibrous capsule around the device is well established. A two-stage approach makes less sense for a patient with coexisting cataract. If the GDD is not connected at the time of cataract surgery, it cannot provide any protection against IOP spikes in the immediate postoperative period.

STEP-BY-STEP PROCEDURE (TWO-SITE GDD AND PHACOEMULSIFICATION)

First, a retrobulbar or peribulbar block is given. Following this, the patient is prepped and draped, and a lid speculum. A closed blade or 'double wired' speculum may provide a better fulcrum for a traction suture.

CONJUNCTIVAL DISSECTION

To begin with, the best quadrant for GDD placement must be selected. The superotemporal site is most suited for large implants and a direct surgical approach, but should be avoided if extensive conjunctival or scleral abnormalities exist. Balloon the conjunctiva with balanced salt solution (BSS) or lidocaine in a 30-gauge needle or manipulate it with a cellulose sponge to identify areas of conjunctival adhesion, if needed to aid with site selection. An adjacent site for the cataract incision is selected from either side of the quadrant where the shunt is placed, adjusting the stool and microscope to comfortably accommodate the approach. The surgeon can choose either a superior or a temporal clear or near-clear corneal incision. In eyes with extensive superior scarring, the shunt can be placed in the inferotemporal quadrant combined with a temporal clear cornea cataract extraction. The higher risk of infection seen with inferior filtering blebs following trabeculectomy is not seen with inferior GDDs, although diplopia and lower lid abnormalities are more commonly encountered.

A traction suture may be placed in the rectus muscle or cornea. When doing a corneal traction suture, 50% depth is optimal; a full thickness corneal pass will cause progressive hypotony as the case continues. Next, a conjunctival peritomy is done in the quadrant selected for GDD placement. The peritomy should be at least 3 to 4 clock hours long, with small relaxing incisions at one or both ends. Blunt dissection with Westcott and/or Stevens scissors is done to create a large sub-Tenon's scleral bed for the drainage device plate. The surgeon needs to dissect as posteriorly as possible so that the implant will be positioned away from the limbus. The surgeon should use nontoothed forceps to hold the conjunctiva to prevent buttonholes. The identification of the adjacent rectus muscles may help the surgeon avoid cutting muscle fibers or the muscle insertion. Achieving hemostasis with cautery of the scleral bed is important, although it is not recommended to cauterize the conjunctival edge.

PLACEMENT OF GDD

Before the device is sutured to the sclera, the surgeon should check its patency by irrigating the tube with a 27-gauge cannula connected to a syringe with BSS. This is mandatory with the Ahmed valve. Soaking the device in an antibiotic solution prior to

fixation to the sclera is optional. If the GDD does not fit into the prepared sub-Tenon's pocket easily, or seems to migrate anteriorly, further dissection or redirection of the implant may be required. The edges of the plate can lie either above or under the rectus muscles. A double-plate Molteno or Ahmed implant can be placed in two adjacent quadrants, with the connecting tube, either under or over the intervening rectus muscle. When positioned, the most anterior aspect of the plate should be at least 8–10 mm posterior to the limbus (Figures 8.1–8.3). There should not be excessive posterior force from Tenon's capsule or adhesions pushing the shunt forward.

If posterior pressure exists, the surgeon should remove the GDD and extend the posterior dissection of the sub-Tenon's space to an adequate size. If a small buttonhole is created, it can be repaired with 8-0 Vicryl suture. If a large buttonhole is created, the quadrant may need to be abandoned for an alternative site. Watertight closure of the primary site should be achieved before starting a new peritomy elsewhere. When the shunt position is considered satisfactory, anchor it to the underlying sclera with Mersilene or nylon sutures tied in a 3-1-1 fashion. Lastly, the surgeon lays the tube onto the cornea and estimates how long the tube should

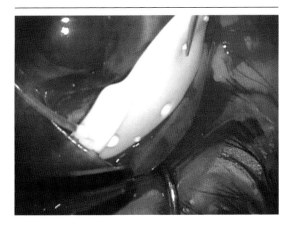

Figure 8.1 The plate is inserted into the prepared quadrant.

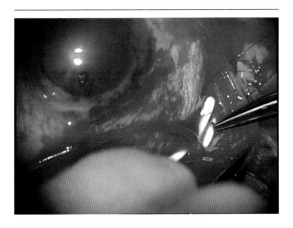

Figure 8.2 The plate is sewn into position, several millimeters posterior to the limbus.

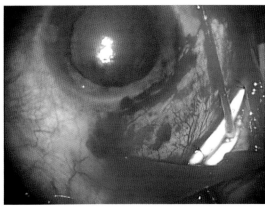

Figure 8.3 The plate sewn into position.

be to extend 2–3 mm beyond the limbus into the anterior chamber (Figure 8.4). Take care not to stretch the tube whilst estimating its length. We use straight scissors to trim a bevel-up end and then turn our attention to the cataract extraction.

PHACOEMULSIFICATION

After adjusting the stools and microscope for a clear or near-clear corneal incision, the surgeon should release or adjust the traction suture to rotate the eye to an optimal position. The paracentesis is placed away from both the planned cataract incision and shunt entry site. The anterior chamber is inflated with viscoelastic (air/indocyanine green/nonpreserved lidocaine optional). The usual clear or near-clear cornea incision is created with a keratome (Figure 8.5). A capsulorhexis is made with a cystotome and/or Utrata forceps. The surgeon then proceeds with hydrodissection/hydrodelineation with BSS, division/removal of the nucleus with the phacoemulsification handpiece and chopper/cracker of choice, and cortical remnant removal with irrigation/aspiration (Figures 8.6 and 8.7). The capsular bag and chamber are then inflated with viscoelastic and the intraocular lens is inserted (Figure 8.8). The viscoelastic is then removed only if it contains particulates/debris. The anterior chamber is hyperinflated with viscoelastic, pushing

the iris away from the cornea and opening the angle as widely as possible (Figure 8.9). The corneal incision is hydrated and/or sutured so that a watertight closure is obtained.

INSERTION OF GDD TUBE INTO THE ANTERIOR CHAMBER

Using a 23-gauge needle on the viscoelastic syringe, the surgeon inserts the needle 2–3 mm posterior to the limbus and tracks it through the sclera so that it emerges in the anterior chamber angle and avoids

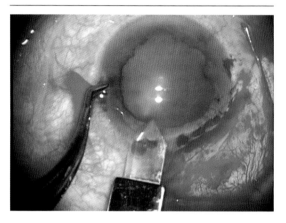

Figure 8.5 The tube is pushed aside to begin cataract surgery. The cataract incision is made some distance away from the planned tube entry site.

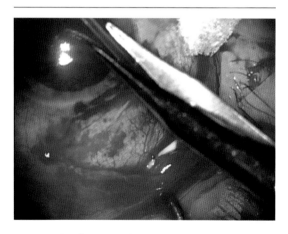

Figure 8.4 The tube is trimmed in a beveled fashion to an appropriate length.

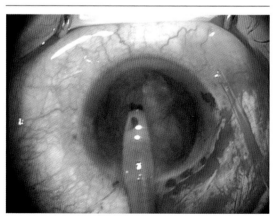

Figure 8.6 Standard phacoemulsification of the nucleus.

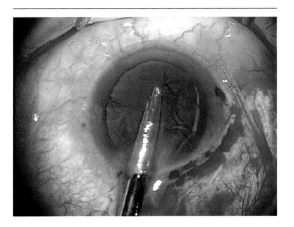

Figure 8.7 Irrigation and aspiration of cortical material.

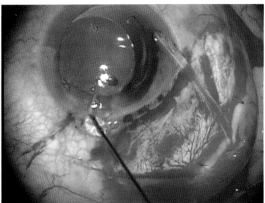

Figure 8.9 The intraocular lens is centered and the anterior chamber is filled with viscoelastic.

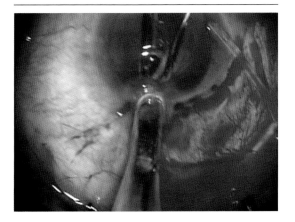

Figure 8.8 Insertion of the intraocular lens.

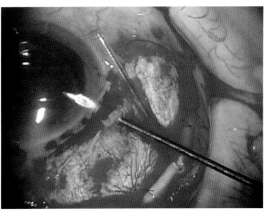

Figure 8.10 A 23-gauge needle is used to create a tract from behind the limbus through the angle into the chamber.

both cornea and iris (Figure 8.10). It helps to make the course of the needle parallel to the natural position of the tube. Once the needle is completely inserted, it is slowly withdrawn while injecting viscoelastic. As the bevel of the needle reaches the outer sclera, the tip of the needle is used to slice slightly to one side. Making the entrance wound larger in this manner facilitates insertion of the tube. If there are extensive peripheral synechiae or if the patient is aphakic, the surgeon may opt to insert the tube just behind the iris or directly through the pars plana into the posterior chamber.

The tube is then prepared for insertion. If it does not have a valve-like mechanism, an absorbable suture can be tied around the silicone tube, or a larger absorbable suture can be placed into the lumen of the tube. Alternatively, a nonabsorbable suture can be tied around (it can be cut with the argon laser postoperatively) or a larger nonabsorbable suture can be left in the tube lumen. This suture is externalized through the cornea or conjunctiva. It can be pulled out with forceps at an appropriate time in the postoperative period. Once the tube has been ligated or occluded, it is guided through the needle tract (Figure 8.11); it should lie flat and not touch the cornea and/or be entrapped by the iris. The surgeon can redirect the tube, if necessary, until the position is felt to be satisfactory (Figure 8.12).

PLACEMENT OF PATCH GRAFT

A patch graft should be placed over the entrance site of the tube into the sclera as well as the exposed area of the tube in front of the plate. Graft tissue can be donor sclera, pericardium (Figure 8.13), dura mater, or fascia lata. This tissue should be trimmed to an approximate 3 × 5–7 mm size. The size of the patch graft can be modified after it is placed over the tube. Cutting off the corners of a square or rectangular graft can facilitate the surgeon's suturing the graft. Three or four interrupted nylon or polyglactin sutures at the corners will usually suffice to hold the patch graft in place.

CLOSURE OF CONJUNCTIVAL WOUND

It is important to lightly deepithelialize the limbal area in order to encourage adhesion of the conjunctival edge. The surgeon should attempt to advance the conjunctiva well over the plate and should try to eliminate as much tension on the tissue as possible. The conjunctiva can be tightly closed into the prepared limbal bed with two anchoring 8-0 Vicryl sutures that are sewn in a running, nonlocking fashion (Figure 8.14). If desired, additional BSS or viscoelastic can be injected through the paracentesis to firm the globe and to help prevent initial hypotony. Subconjunctival injections of steroid and/or antibiotics are optional, although subconjunctival solumedrol or kenalog is especially helpful in cases of inflammatory glaucoma (Figures 8.15 and 8.16). At the end of the case, the eye is lightly pressure patched for 12–24 hours.

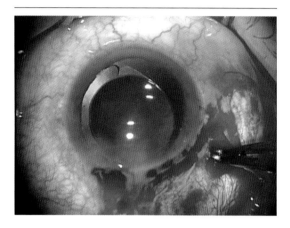

Figure 8.11 The tube is inserted into the tract opening.

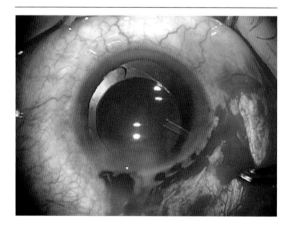

Figure 8.12 The tube length is checked after insertion is complete. If it encroaches on the visual axis, it can be trimmed and reinserted.

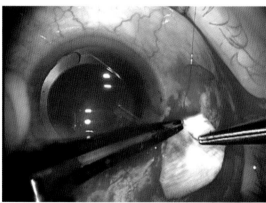

Figure 8.13 A pericardial tissue graft is sewn over the exposed tube with interrupted sutures.

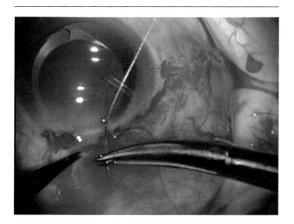

Figure 8.14 Conjunctiva and Tenon's are brought forward to the limbus and sewn in a watertight fashion with running suture.

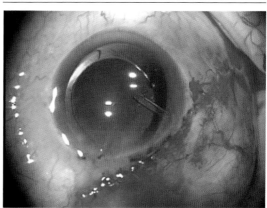

Figure 8.16 Shunt in good position with watertight closure at the end of the case.

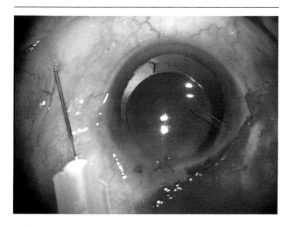

Figure 8.15 Subconjunctival injections are administered.

coelastic. A keratome is used to create a full-thickness entry into the anterior chamber through the scleral tunnel.

Phacoemulsifcation is performed as previously described. The trimmed tube is then inserted through the scleral tunnel into the anterior chamber; it is important to secure the scleral tunnel as tightly as possible around the tube. Tube ligatures to prevent hypotony are even more critical in this situation because of the additional flow around the tube through the tunnel. Additional biograft material may not be necessary if there is already adequate coverage of the tube by the scleral tunnel.

ONE-SITE PROCEDURE WITH SCLERAL-TUNNEL PHACOEMULSIFICATION

Initially, the external device is attached to the globe in a fashion similar to the two-site technique. A scleral tunnel is then created immediately anterior to the external GDD. A partial-thickness scleral incision 3.0–3.5 mm in length is created 2 to 3 mm posterior and parallel to the limbus. The 69-Beaver cleft palate blade is used to dissect the tunnel into clear cornea. After tne scleral tunnel is created, a paracentesis is done and the eye is filled with vis-

ONE-SITE APPROACH USING A LARGE INCISION FOR EXTRACAPSULAR CATARACT EXTRACTION

After the GDD is sewn to the external globe as described above, a 10–12 mm conjunctival peritomy at the limbus is required. A small diamond or ruby blade can then be used to make a partial-thickness limbal groove. Then a paracentesis is created in the groove and the anterior chamber is deepened with viscoelastic. Following this, a keratome is used to create a full-thickness entry into the anterior chamber through the groove.

A capsulorhexis or postage-stamp capsulotomy is performed with a cystotome and/or Utrata forceps, and hydrodissection with BSS is performed. The full-thickness incision is then extended to the entire 8–10 mm length of the groove with the keratome or corneal scissors. At this point, two 10-0 nylon sutures are passed through the 10 o'clock and 2 o'clock positions in the incision. They should be left long and loose to allow room for the nucleus.

Using Kelman-McPherson forceps at the 6 o'clock position and a lens loop at the 12 o'clock position, the surgeon places gentle pressure first at 6 then at 12 o'clock and then simultaneously to encourage delivery of the nucleus. An assistant can pick up the corneal edge of the wound to aid in the lens delivery. Once the nucleus is out, the preplaced corneal sutures are tied. Irrigation/aspiration of cortex is performed, the bag is inflated with viscoelastic, and the lens implant is placed in the capsular bag. The incision is closed with an adequate number of interrupted or running 10-0 nylon sutures, and the chamber is deepened with viscoelastic.

At this point, the surgeon can either place the tube shunt through the limbal cataract incision between two sutures, or create a more posterior tract for the shunt using a 23-gauge needle. The latter is far preferable, since it will keep the tube angled farther away from the cornea. The more anterior the cataract incision is, the greater the chances of the tube abutting the corneal endothelium and causing permanent decompensation. There is also increased difficulty getting a patch graft and adequate conjunctival covering over an anterior tube entry point. If the patient has been left aphakic or with an anterior chamber intraocular lens, an adequate vitrectomy should be performed. The tube can then be introduced through pars plana to lie in the posterior chamber.

INTRAOPERATIVE HAZARDS/COMPLICATIONS

RETROBULBAR HEMORRHAGE/GLOBE PERFORATION

GDD procedures are best performed under sedation and a retrobulbar block or general anesthesia. Precautions to avoid retrobulbar hemorrhage are prudent, especially in predisposed patients. Pharmacological anticoagulation should be reduced preoperatively if there are no contraindications. In high-risk anticoagulated patients, the block could be modified to peribulbar. Supplementation with intracameral nonpreserved lidocaine is optional.

INADVERTENT GLOBE PERFORATION WITH SUTURES

Immediate retinal consultation is advisable if a full thickness scleral penetration posterior to pars plana is suspected.

CONJUNCTIVAL BUTTONHOLES

All conjunctival closures should be watertight at the end of the case. If conjunctival closures have microleaks due to poor tissue quality, extended pressure patching may allow secondary healing.

INADEQUATE AMOUNT OF CONJUNCTIVAL TISSUE

A rotational or free conjunctival graft may be required to adequately cover the device and patch graft. It is advisable not to place a free flap over the device itself, as it will likely fail without underlying tissue.

EXPULSIVE HEMORRHAGE

Be aware of patients at high risk for intraoperative choroidal hemorrhage. Risk factors include glaucoma (especially with uncontrolled IOP), advanced age, frail health, and anticoagulants. Meaures to decrease anticoagulation may be taken preoperatively if not otherwise contraindicated. When initially entering the eye, allow for a slow removal of aqueous through the paracentesis rather than rapid decompression.

CAPSULAR RUPTURE

An exhaustive discussion of capsular rupture is beyond the scope of this text. If vitreous is encountered, an adequate vitrectomy must be performed to prevent a later tractional detachment or blockage of the GDD tip with vitreous. In the event of a capsular break, one should attempt to preserve anterior capsular rim for placement of a posterior chamber IOL in the sulcus. Consider modifying tip placement to pars plana if the patient must be left aphakic or with an anterior chamber intraocular lens. In this event, subtotal vitrectomy is advisable.

POSTOPERATIVE COMPLICATIONS

HYPERTENSIVE PHASE/SHUNT FAILURE

Most eyes experience a significant IOP rise about 2–4 weeks after GDD placement. This spike may be due to loss of flow around the outside of the device tube, and to the tight fibrous capsule around the GDD plate. IOP may return to preoperative levels or higher. This phase may last several weeks to a few months, or even longer. As the capsule matures and collagen changes occur, the IOP will drift back down. It may be desirable to resume some or all of the preoperative medications during the hypertensive phase. One-fourth to one-half of eyes will require supplemental medications indefinitely.

CORNEAL ENDOTHELIAL COMPROMISE

The intraocular portion of the tube should lie flat in the anterior chamber, well away from the cornea. If the chamber shallows in the postoperative period, supplemental viscoelastic can be added through the paracentesis to push the tube back from the cornea. A mattress suture can also be placed to hold the tip more posteriorly.

RELEASABLE SUTURES

Temporary ligatures can be a source of discomfort and a potential route for intraocular infection. If either becomes a concern, it may be necessary to remove the suture material, even if there is persistent hypotony.

HYPOTONY

Many eyes go through at least a 2–3 week period of transient hypotony following the procedure, especially if no tube-occluding suture is placed. Temporary ligatures and intracameral viscoelastic may be used to prevent severe low pressure. Aggressive use of anti-inflammatory agents and cycloplegia can help break the cycle of inflammation/ciliary shutdown/hypotony/choroidal effusion that can often be seen following glaucoma surgery.

WOUND LEAK

Very small limbal wound leaks will sometimes resolve spontaneously. It is recommended to lightly pressure patch with ointment for 24–48 hours. Larger leaks will require additional sutures. A chronic eroded area may require further modification, with additional patch graft material and extensive conjunctival revision. It is difficult to successfully graft any tissue over the drainage device plate; it will usually erode again in a short time. It may be necessary to explant the device.

TUBE OCCLUSION

Transient tube occlusion with blood, inflammatory debris, pigment, or viscoelastic may occur in the immediate postoperative period. If not severe, it can usually be observed until the fibrin retracts and the occlusion spontaneously resolves. During the late postoperative period, clogs at the shunt tip may be disrupted using a YAG laser.

TUBE EXTRUSION

If the tube extrudes from the anterior chamber because of inadequate length, additional material may be spliced to the tip prior to repositioning. A flexible silastic catheter can be attached to the existing tube with cyanoacrylate adhesive.

MOTILITY DISORDERS

The GDD plate and capsule can infringe upon adjacent rectus muscles, inducing motility disturbances. Patients with adequate visual acuity may experience diplopia. Spreading the filtration area into two quadrants by using a double plate Molteno device may decrease the incidence of strabismus. Symptoms usually improve over time.

INFECTIONS

The incidence of endophthalmitis following GDD is very low. It is recommended that patients continue topical antibiotic drops for at least 10–14 days after surgery. Patients with wound leaks should have antibiotic coverage until the leak has completely resolved.

EPITHELIAL INGROWTH

Epithelial ingrowth can occur in the face of wound leak, chronic hypotony, and inflammation following ocular surgery or trauma. Careful wound construction and vigilant postoperative care should help minimize the risk for this dreaded complication, which may be difficult or impossible to eradicate, once established.

SPECIAL SITUATIONS

NARROW ANGLE GLAUCOMA

Patients with hyperopia and narrow angle or primary angle closure glaucoma present additional challenges. Inflammation and corneal edema may accompany an acute closure attack. Patients with large cataracts may have a phacomorphic component. Cataract extraction may be more difficult due to posterior pressure and shallow chamber. The surgeon's view can be improved by reducing corneal edema with glycerine. Aggressive preoperative IOP lowering with the Honan balloon and/or systemic carbonic anhydrase inhibitors can be helpful. Tube insertion can also be challenging. The surgeon should try to open the angle as widely as possible with viscoelastic to allow good tube placement. If the iris has been damaged by ischemia, dilation may be poor.

TRAUMA

When there is a history of previous trauma, the surgeon needs to be particularly alert for any zonular instability. Angle synechiae can interfere with tube placement.

DIABETES AND/OR NEOVASCULAR GLAUCOMA

GDDs may have a marginally better success rate than trabeculectomy with antimetabolites in patients with rubeosis and neovascular glaucoma. The GDDs may be particularly useful with florid neovascularization, since it is not necessary to perform a surgical iridectomy during shunt implantation, and fibrous membranes do not adhere well to the tube. Florid iris neovascularization makes cataract extraction extremely challenging.

MONOCULAR PATIENT

A combined cataract and drainage procedure is particularly attractive when the patient's only seeing eye is affected with both cataract and uncontrolled glaucoma. The patient should understand that a combined procedure does carry a higher risk than either procedure performed alone.

UVEITIS

Shunt devices are a good way to stabilize these patients who may be prone to wide IOP fluctuations, and in whom standard trabeculectomies are prone to scar.

CONCLUSION

Combined cataract and GDD procedures have a role in the management of the glaucoma patient with a coexisting, visually significant cataract.

FURTHER READING

Azuara-Blanco A, Moster MR, Wilson RP, Schmidt CM. Simultaneous use of mitomycin-C with Baerveldt implantation. Ophthalmic Surg Lasers 1997; 28: 992–7.

Ball SF, Herrington RG. Long-term retention of chromic occlusion suture in glaucoma seton tubes. Arch Ophthalmol 1993; 111: 169.

Brandt JD. Patch grafts of dehydrated cadaveric dura mater for tube-shunt glaucoma surgery. Arch Ophthalmol 1993; 111: 1436.

Britt MT, LaBree LD, Lloyd MA et al. Randomized clinical trial of the 340-mm² versus the 500-mm² Baerveldt implant; longer term results: is bigger better? Ophthalmology 1999; 106: 2312–18.

Camras CB et al. Valved tube shunt from the anterior chamber to the external ocular surface for use in refractory glaucoma. Invest Ophthalmol Vis Sci 1992; 33(suppl): 949.

Cantor L, Burgoyne J, Sanders S, Bhavnani V, Hoop J, Brizendine E. The effect of mitomycin C on Molteno implant surgery; a 1-year randomized, masked, prospective study. J Glaucoma 1998; 7: 240–6.

Cashwell LF, Shields MB. Surgical management of coexisting cataract and glaucoma. In: Ritch R, Shields MB, Krupin T, eds. The Glaucomas: St Louis: Mosby-Year Book, 1996: 1745–59.

Coleman AL, Hill R, Wilson MR et al. Initial clinical experience with the Ahmed glaucoma valve implant. Am J Ophthalmol 1995; 120: 23–31

Desatnik HR, Foster RE, Rockwood EJ et al. Management of glaucoma implants occluded by vitreous incarceration. J Glaucoma 2000; 9: 311–16.

Dobler-Dixon AA, Cantor LB, Sondhi N, Ku WS, Hoop J. Prospective evaluation of extraocular motility following double-plate Molteno implantation. Arch Ophthalmol 1999; 117: 1155–60.

Egbert PR, Lieberman MF. Internal suture occlusion of the Molteno glaucoma implant for the prevention of postoperative hypotony. Ophthalmic Surg 1989; 20: 53.

El-Sayad F el-Maghraby A, Helal M, Amayem A. The use of releasable sutures in Molteno glaucoma implant procedures to reduce postoperative hypotony. Ophthalmic Surg 1991; 22: 82.

Fiore PM, Melamed S. Use of neodymium:YAG laser to open an occluded Molteno tube. Ophthalmic Surg 1989; 20: 201.

Fitzgerald-Shelton K, Higginbotham EJ. Comparison of the Baerveldt implant with the double-plate Molteno implant. Arch Ophthalmol 1996; 114: 1030; discussion 1031.

Gedde SJ, Scott IU, Tabandeh H et al. Late endophthalmitis associated with glaucoma drainage implants. Ophthalmology 2001; 108: 1323–7.

Greenfield DS, Tello C, Budenz DL, Liebmann JM, Ritch R. Aqueous misdirection after glaucoma drainage device implantation. Ophthalmology 1999; 106: 1035–40.

Hodkin MJ, Goldblatt WS, Burgoyne CF, Ball SF, Insler MS. Early clinical experience with the Baerveldt implant in complicated glaucoma. Am J Ophthalmol 1995; 120: 32.

Joos KM, Lavina AM, Tawansy KA, Aggarwal A. Posterior repositioning of glaucoma implants for anterior segment complications. Ophthalmology 2001; 108: 279–84.

Krebs DB, Liebmann JM, Ritch R, Speaker M. Late infectious endophthalmitis from exposed glaucoma setons. Arch Ophthalmol 1992; 110: 174.

Krishna R, Godfrey DG, Budenz DL et al. Intermediate-term outcomes of 350-mm² Baerveldt glaucoma implants. Ophthalmology 2001; 108: 621–6.

Latina MA. Single stage Molteno implant with combination internal occlusion and external ligature. Ophthalmic Surg 1990; 21: 444.

Liebmann JM, Ritch R. Intraocular suture ligature to reduce hypotony following Molteno seton implantation. Ophthalmic Surg 1992; 23: 51.

Lotufo DG. Postoperative complications and visual loss following Molteno implantation. Ophthalmic Surg 1991; 22: 650.

Lloyd M, Heuer DK, Baerveldt G, et al. Combined Molteno implantation and pars plana vitrectomy for neovascular glaucoma. Ophthalmology 1991; 98: 1401.

Lloyd ME, Baerveldt G, Heuer DK, Minckler DS, Martone JF. Initial clinical experience with the Baerveldt implant in complicated glaucomas. Ophthalmology 1994; 101: 640.

Lloyd ME, Baerveldt G, Tellenbaum PS, et al. Intermediate-term results of a randomized clinical trial of the 350 mm² vs. the 500 mm² Baerveldt implant. Ophthalmology 1994; 101: 1456.

Luttrull JK, Avery RL, Baerveldt G, Easley KA. Initial experience with pneumatically stented Baerveldt implant modified for pars plana insertion for complicated glaucoma. Ophthalmology 2000; 107: 143–9; discussion 149–50.

McCartney DL, Memmen YE, Stark WY, Quigley HA, Maumenee AE, Gottsch YD. The efficacy and safety of combined trabeculectomy, cataract extraction and intraocular lens implantation. Ophthalmology 1998; 95: 754.

McDermott ML, Swendris RP, Shin DH, Juzych MS, Cowden JW. Corneal endothelial cell counts after Molteno implantation. Am J Ophthalmol 1993; 115: 93.

McQueen BR, Margo CE. Capsular bag distention syndrome after combined cataract-lens implant surgery and Ahmed valve implantation. Am J Ophthalmol 2001; 132: 109–10.

Melamed S, Cahane M, Gutman I, Blumenthal M. Postoperative complications after Molteno implant surgery. Am J Ophthalmol 1991; 111: 319.

Mermoud A, Salmon JF, Alexander P, Straker C, Murray AD. Molteno tube implantation for neovascular glaucoma; long-term results and factors influencing outcome. Ophthalmology 1993; 100: 897.

Minckler DS, Shammas A, Wilcox M, Ogden TE. Experimental studies of aqueous filtration using the Molteno implant. Trans Am Ophthalmol Soc 1987; 85: 368–92.

Minckler DS, Heuer DK, Hasty B, et al. Clinical experience with the single-plate Molteno implant in complicated glaucoma. Ophthalmology 1998; 95: 1181–8.

Netland PA, Walton DS. Glaucoma drainage implants in pediatric patients. Ophthalmic Surg 1993; 24: 723.

Nguyen QH, Budenz DL, Parrish RK II. Complications of Baerveldt glaucoma drainage implants. Arch Ophthalmol 1998; 116: 571–5.

Pastor SA, Schumann SP, Starita RJ, Fellman RL. Intracameral tissue plasminogen activator: management of a fibrin clot occluding a Molteno tube. Ophthalmic Surg 1993; 24: 853.

Perkins TW, Cardakli UF, Eisele JR, Kaufman PL, Heatley GA. Adjunctive mitomycin C in Molteno implant surgery. Ophthalmology 1995; 102: 91.

Prata JA Jr, Mermoud A, LeBree L, Minckler DS. In-vitro and in-vivo flow characteristics of glaucoma drainage implants. Ophthalmology 1995; 102: 894–904.

Rhee DJ, Casuso LA, Rosa RH Jr, Budenz DL. Motility disturbance due to true Tenon cyst in a child with a Baerveldt glaucoma drainage implant. Arch Ophthalmol 2001; 119: 440–2.

Rosenberg LF, Krupin T. Implants in glaucoma surgery. In: Ritch R, Shields MB, Krupin T, eds: The Glaucomas. 2nd edn. St. Louis: Mosby-Year Book, 1996: 1783–1807.

Shepherd DM. The pupil stretch technique for miotic pupils in cataract surgery. Ophthalmic Surg 1993; 24: 851.

Sherwood MB, Smith MF. Prevention of early hypotony associated with Molteno implants by a new occluding stent technique. Ophthalmology 1993; 100: 85.

Shields MB. Another reevaluation of combined cataract and glaucoma surgery. Am J Ophthalmol 1993; 115: 806.

Trible JR, Brown DB. Occlusive ligature and standardized fenestration of a Baerveldt tube with and without antimetabolites for early postoperative intraocular pressure control. Ophthalmology 1998; 105: 2243–50.

9. Combined cataract–nonpenetrating glaucoma surgery

Tarek Shaarawy, Fathi El-Sayyad and André Mermoud

INTRODUCTION

Technologic advances in the surgical management of glaucoma and cataract have expanded the potential options for the effective management of these two conditions. However, the management choices still include three basic surgical approaches: cataract extraction followed by glaucoma surgery, glaucoma filtering surgery alone with a later cataract extraction, and combined cataract–glaucoma surgery.

Combined surgical management of coexisting cataract and glaucoma has gained popularity because of several advantages, which include decreased risk and easier management of early postoperative intraocular pressure (IOP) spikes, better long-term glaucoma control with respect to IOP and/or medications, and the need to perform only one surgical procedure to manage both the cataract and chronic glaucoma.

The technologic innovations of small-incision cataract surgery have changed the outcome of the combined procedure in those eyes with coexisting cataract and glaucoma. Phacoemulsification with a glaucoma operation provides IOP control comparable with two-stage surgery (glaucoma surgery followed by cataract extraction) and has the additional advantages of requiring only one operation with earlier visual rehabilitation.

Although trabeculectomy is currently considered the standard surgical procedure combined with cataract surgery, it is associated with potentially vision-threatening complications including hyphema, excessive filtration leading to shallow or flat anterior chamber, choroidal detachments, hypotony maculopathy, suprachoroidal hemorrhage bleb-related problems and increased risk of endophthalmitis.

Nonpentrating glaucoma surgery (NPGS) is an alternative to trabeculectomy and has the advantage of decreased early postoperative complications. In comparative studies, postoperative IOP control was statistically similar in combined procedures with a trabeculectomy versus those with NPGS than with combined trabeculectomies. The recent advances of NPGS with phacoemulsification surgery and its satisfactory results regarding visual outcome and IOP control have made the option of combined cataract and glaucoma surgery quite appealing to both patients and surgeons alike.

SURGICAL TECHNIQUE

Topical anesthesia can be used in combined viscocanalostomy or deep sclerectomy and phacoemulsification (bupivacaine (5%) eye drops). It is relatively comfortable because a peripheral iridectomy is not needed during the nonpenetrating procedure. Alternatively, a retrobulbar injection of 3–6 ml of a bupivacaine (0.75%), lidocaine (2%) and hyaluronidase (50 U) solution can be used.

Box 9.1 gives the list of instruments required. A 7-0 superior peripheral corneal silk or Vicryl suture is used for traction. This is more convenient than a superior rectus traction suture, especially if topical anesthesia is used. In addition, it eliminates the risk of a subconjunctival hemorrhage, a buttonhole and postoperative ptosis that can result from a bridle suture.

The combined procedure can be performed two ways: (i) a shared or one-site incision through which the deep sclerectomy and phacoemulsification are performed, or (ii) a clear corneal incision for the phacoemulsification which is separate from the deep sclerectomy site. We prefer the two-site technique with a temporal incision for the

Box 9.1 List of surgical instruments

7-0 traction suture
Nontoothed forceps
Vasopressin
Weck cell sponges
Cautery
Grieshaber minispoon blade
Diamond knife
Viscoelastic
Vannas scissors
Special forceps (Huco vision SA, ST Blaise, Switzerland)
Grishhaber cannula
Collagen implant (Staar, Nidau, Switerland)
Reticulated hyaluronic acid (Corneal, France)
Nylon sutures

phacoemulsification and a 12 o'clock site for the deep sclerectomy. We hypothesize that a two-site approach is associated with a more stable wound, and has fewer instances of membrane perforation, although, to the best of our knowledge, this has not been systematically studied.

An 8–9 mm wide, fornix-based conjunctival flap is prepared in the desired location usually superiorly. Alternatively, the conjunctiva and Tenon's capsule are opened in the upper fornix and the sclera is exposed. A fornix-based flap may be preferred, since it is simpler, gives better exposure during phacoemulsification and fashioning of the superficial and deep scleral flaps, and is easier to close (Figure 9.1).

Minimal but careful coagulation is advisable to preserve the function of episcleral vessels for aqueous drainage in the deep sclerectomy procedure. A vasopressin-soaked Weck cell sponge may be applied to bleeders to aid hemostasis. Light cautery also avoids excessive scarring and retraction of the scleral tissue. Different shapes and dimensions of superficial sclera flaps have been described in combined surgery. A larger flap may be hypothetically favoured in order to increase the surface area of drainage when the deeper scleral flap is excised.

CREATING THE SCLERAL FLAP

The scleral flap is fashioned between collector channels and the shape is usually a square measuring 5×5 mm (Figure 9.2). The outline of the superficial flap is made 300 μm deep (roughly one third of scleral thickness), then planar dissection starts at the posterior angle and advances forward using a Huco vision ruby knife (Figure 9.3) (St Blaise, Switzerland) or Grieshaber mini spoon blade (Schaffhausen, Switzerland). It is important to preserve the integrity of the superficial flap and to avoid shredding it since conversion to trabeculectomy may be required.

The blade, which is held parallel to the scleral flap, is advanced forward with light pressure against the scleral bed. As the knife is held parallel and advanced forward, dissection takes place with the whole edge of the knife, thus ensuring an even

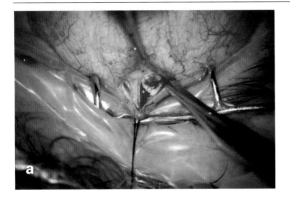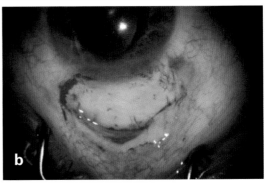

Figure 9.1 (a) A limbal-based conjunctival incision. (b) Fornix-based conjunctival incision.

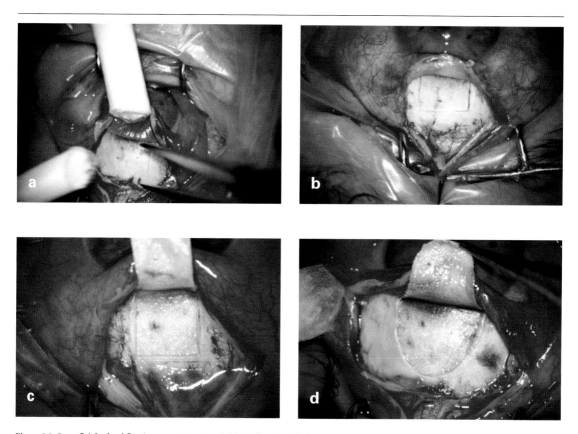

Figure 9.2 Superficial scleral flap (measures 5 × 5 mm). (a) Application of light cantery to bleeding vessels. (b) Delineation of superficial scleral flap with metal blade, depth of incision about 300 μm. (c) Extension of superficial scleral flap into clear cornea for 1–1.5 mm. (d) Variation in shape of superficial scleral flap.

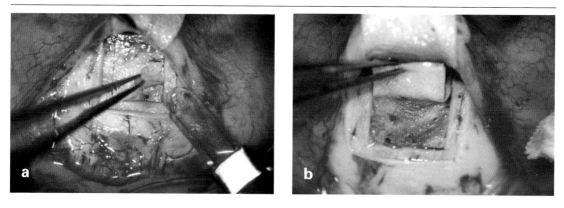

Figure 9.3 (a) Beginning of a deep sclerotomy horizontal dissection with a ruby blade. (b) Horizontal dissection in progress at halfway stage.

dissection. If the knife is held at an angle, there will be an uneven dissection of the flap. The flap is dissected for 1 mm into clear cornea.

PHACOEMULSIFICATION

Phacoemulsification is usually done before the deep flap dissection as the irrigation pressure could rupture the fragile trabeculo-Descemet's membrane (TDM). If the deeper flap is dissected first, we do not recommend advancing into clear cornea before phacoemulsification. After the cataract is removed, the surgeon can complete and excise the deeper flap.

A temporal incision in clear cornea is performed with a diamond knife (Figure 9.4). Viscoelastic material is then introduced and a paracentesis is performed (Figure 9.5) to allow bimanual phacoemulsification. After anterior capsulorhexis and hydrodissection, the lens nucleus is removed by phacoemulsification and the remaining cortex is removed by manual irrigation and aspiration. The incision is then widened to 4 mm and a foldable intraocular lens is introduced into the capsular bag. The temporal incision is usually left sutureless, and the surgeon should proceed to finishing the deep sclerectomy dissection.

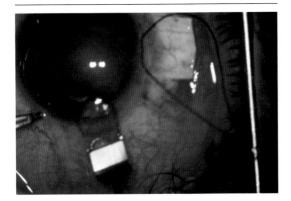

Figure 9.4 Separate-site phacoemulsification incision through temporal cornea.

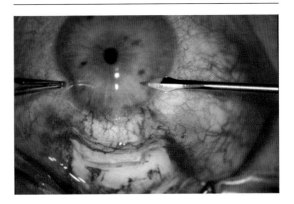

Figure 9.5 Paracentesis.

CREATING THE DEEPER FLAP

A 4 × 4 mm square deeper scleral flap is fashioned under the superficial one and the dissection is started as near as possible to the choroid. Uveal tissue glistening through the very thin scleral layer should be seen. A useful hint is to dissect deep enough until the choroid is identified and exposed at the posterior angle of the deep flap. Full dissection of the deeper flap is then done just above the level of the choroid. No complications have been reported from exposure of a small amount of choroid. It is important to do the dissection in a plane of sufficient depth in order to unroof Schlemm's canal. The dissection is advanced anteriorly, unroofing Schlemm's canal. The canal appears as a darker line anterior to the scleral spur.

The dissection of the deep scleral flap is continued towards the limbus to expose the sclerocorneal trabecular meshwork. The dissection is extended 1 mm into clear cornea (Figure 9.6). Blunt dissection with gentle pressure just anterior to Schlemm's canal using a sponge is used to detach Descemet's membrane from the corneal stroma, creating a Descemet's window. It is well advised to have a wide window (1–2 mm) which might facilitate Nd:YAG gonipuncture if the IOP increases postoperatively. The deeper flap is excised using a diamond knife or Vannas scissors after achieving adequate aqueous percolation through the TDM.

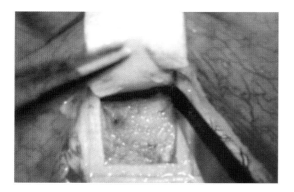

Figure 9.6 Radial cut with metal blade held upside down to expose Descemet's membrane.

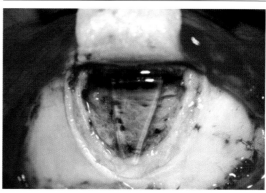

Figure 9.7 SK gel.

The juxtacanalicular trabecular membrane and the inner wall of Schlemm's canal are peeled off using a special forceps (Huco vision). At this stage, aqueous humor can be seen percolating through the remaining TDM. If percolation is inadequate, further peeling is needed. Care should be taken to avoid perforation of the window.

Recent studies have shown the importance of artificially occuping the surgically created intra-scleral space. In viscocanalostomy, high molecular weight sodium hyaluronate acid (Healon GV, Pharmacia and Upjohn AB, Sweden) is injected into the open ends of Schlemm's canal using a fine cannula (Grieshaber). The high molecular weight viscoelastic is thought to mechanically dilate the lumen of the canal of Schlemm, restoring the physiological outflow pathway of aqueous through the canal and the collector channels. Healon GV is then placed under the external flap before it is sutured with two interrupted 10-0 nylon sutures.

In deep sclerectomy, an implant can be sutured in the scleral bed that either dissolves in 6–9 months (collagen implant, Staar) or 50 days (Figure 9.7) (reticulated hyaluronic acid, Corneal). Recently, other nonabsorbable implants have been introduced (T-FLUX, IOLTECH, France). The external flap is also loosely sutured with two interrupted 10-0 nylon sutures.

The intrascleral space is created to act as a reservoir for the aqueous percolation from the anterior chamber through the thin sclerocorneal trabecular meshwork and Descemet's window. Aqueous flows through the dilated ends of Schlemm's canal into the collector channels and the episcleral veins while the conjunctiva is closed with interrupted nylon sutures.

COMPLICATIONS

The most common complication encountered during viscocanalostomy or deep sclerectomy is the perforation of Descemet's window (Figure 9.8). If a microperforation occurs, this can be disregarded and the surgeon can proceed with no adverse complications. However, if a significant perforation occurs, the procedure may be completed as a phacotrabeculectomy with internal block dissection

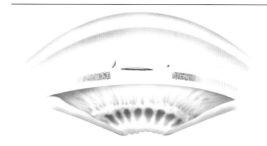

Figure 9.8 Schematric representation of perforation or tear at level of Schwalbe's line as seen by gonioscopy.

and a peripheral iridectomy (for detailed management see Chapters 6 and 7). The surgical outcome of patients undergoing sclerectomy with accidental perforation and conversion to trabeculectomy was analyzed by Sanchez and coworkers who found that the long-term success rate of those eyes was comparable to trabeculectomy. Failure to identify Schlemm's canal is most commonly due to inadequate deep dissection. The surgeon has to start the deeper dissection 2–3 mm posterior to the scleral spur to be able to identify the canal.

The superficial scleral flap may tear especially if there is a shared incision with a combined phacoemulsification. This requires extra suturing to secure the flap to form the aqueous reservoir in the intrascleral space. Early postoperative complications may also include IOP spikes, iris prolapse through the TDM, transient hypotony, hyphema, and shallow anterior chambers.

The resistance to aqueous outflow through the TDM may increase due to gradual thickening of the membrane. Meticulous dissection of the sclera, Schlemm's canal and the peripheral cornea during surgery decreases the incidence of its progressive thickening. Postoperatively goniopuncture using Nd:YAG laser to disrupt the TDM may be used to convert the sclerectomy into a perforating procedure.

CONCLUSION

Combined NPGS with phacoemulsification appears to be a safe and effective procedure. It is an alternative to combined phacoemulsification with trabeculectomy and deserves further study.

FURTHER READING

Ambresin A, Borruat FX, Mermoud A. Recurrent transient visual loss after deep sclerectomy. Arch.Ophthalmol 2001; 119: 1213–15.

Ates H, Andac K, Uretmen O. Non-penetrating deep sclerectomy and collagen implant surgery in glaucoma patients with advanced field loss. Int Ophthalmol 1999; 23: 123–8.

Bas JM, Goethals MJ. Non-penetrating deep sclerectomy preliminary results. Bull Soc Belge Ophtalmol 1999; 272: 55–9.

Baudouin C. [Deep non-perforating sclerectomy: a bad name for good surgery]. J Fr Ophtalmol 1999; 22: 780.

Bylsma S. Nonpenetrating deep sclerectomy: collagen implant and viscocanalostomy procedures. Int Ophthalmol Clin 1999; 39: 103–19.

Carassa RG, Bettin P, Brancato R. Viscocanalostomy: a pilot study. Acta Ophthalmol Scand Suppl 1998; 227: 51–2.

Carassa RG, Bettin P, Fiori M, Brancato R. Viscocanalostomy: a pilot study. Eur J Ophthalmol 1998; 8: 57–61.

Chiou AG, Mermoud A, Hediguer SE. [Malignant ciliary block glaucoma after deep sclerotomy—ultrasound biomicroscopy imaging]. Klin Monatsbl Augenheilkd 1996; 208: 279–81.

Chiou AG, Mermoud A, Hediguer SE, Schnyder CC, Faggioni R. Ultrasound biomicroscopy of eyes undergoing deep sclerectomy with collagen implant. Br J Ophthalmol 1996; 80: 541–4.

Chiou AG, Mermoud A, Jewelewicz DA. Post-operative inflammation following deep sclerectomy with collagen implant versus standard trabeculectomy. Graefes Arch Clin Exp Ophthalmol 1998; 236: 593–6.

Chiselita D. Non-penetrating deep sclerectomy versus trabeculectomy in primary open-angle glaucoma surgery. Eye 2001; 15: 197–201.

Collignon-Brach J. [Glaucoma and cataract—surgery at two times]. Bull Soc Belge Ophtalmol 1998; 268: 61–8.

Crandall AS. Nonpenetrating filtering procedures: viscocanalostomy and collagen wick. Semin Ophthalmol 1999; 14: 189–95.

Dahan E, Drusedau MU. Nonpenetrating filtration surgery for glaucoma: control by surgery only. J Cataract Refract Surg 2000; 26: 695–701.

Detry-Morel M. Non penetrating deep sclerectomy (NPDS) with SKGEL implant and/or 5-fluorouracil (5-FU). Bull Soc Belge Ophtalmol 2001; 280: 23–32.

Di Staso S, Taverniti L, Genitti G et al. Combined phacoemulsification and deep sclerectomy vs phacoemulsification and trabeculectomy. Acta Ophthalmol Scand Suppl 2000; 78: 59–60.

Dietlein TS, Engels BF, Jacobi PC, Krieglstein GK. Ultrasound biomicroscopic patterns after glaucoma surgery in congenital glaucoma. Ophthalmology 2000; 107: 1200–5.

Dietlein TS, Jacobi PC, Luke C, Krieglstein GK. Morphological variability of the trabecular meshwork in glaucoma patients: implications for non-perforating glaucoma surgery. Br J Ophthalmol 2000; 84: 1354–9.

Dietlein TS, Luke C, Jacobi PC, Konen W, Krieglstein GK. Variability of dissection depth in deep sclerectomy: morphological analysis of the deep scleral flap. Graefes Arch Clin Exp Ophthalmol 2000; 238: 405–9.

Dietlein TS, Luke C, Jacobi PC, Konen W, Krieglstein GK. [Does the dissection depth and thickness of the deep scleral flap affect intraocular pressure after viscocanalostomy? A clinico-pathologic correlation]. Klin Monatsbl Augenheilkd 2001; 218: 168–73.

El Sayyad F, Helal M, El Kholify H, Khalil M, El Maghraby A. Nonpenetrating deep sclerectomy versus trabeculectomy in bilateral primary open-angle glaucoma. Ophthalmology 2000; 107: 1671–4.

Fedorov SN, Ioffe DI, Ronkina TI. [Glaucoma surgery—deep sclerectomy]. Vestn Oftalmol 1982; 6–10.

Galand A. [A proposed variation for glaucoma surgery]. Bull Soc Belge Ophtalmol 2000; Suppl: 87–92.

Gianoli F, Mermoud A. [Cataract-glaucoma combined surgery: comparison between phacoemulsification combined with deep sclerectomy, or trabeculectomy]. Klin Monatsbl Augenheilkd 1997; 210: 256–60.

Gianoli F, Schnyder CC, Bovey E, Mermoud A. Combined surgery for cataract and glaucoma: phacoemulsification and deep sclerectomy compared with phacoemulsification and trabeculectomy. J Cataract Refract Surg 1999; 25: 340–6.

Gimbel HV, Penno EE, Ferensowicz M. Combined cataract surgery, intraocular lens implantation, and viscocanalostomy. J Cataract Refract Surg 1999; 25: 1370–5.

Hamard P, Plaza L, Kopel J, Quesnot S, Hamard H. [Deep nonpenetrating sclerectomy and open angle glaucoma. Intermediate results from the first operated patients]. J Fr Ophtalmol 1999; 22: 25–31.

Hamard P, Sourdille P, Valtot F, Baudouin C. [Evaluation of confocal microscopy in the analysis of the external trabecular membrane during deep nonpenetrating sclerectomy]. J Fr Ophtalmol 2001; 24: 29–35.

Hamel M, Shaarawy T, Mermoud A. Deep sclerectomy with collagen implant in patients with glaucoma and high myopia. J Cataract Refract Surg 2001; 27: 1410–17.

Heisler JM, Venjakob H, von Domarus D, Wirt H. [Long-term results of combined glaucoma and cataract surgery. Intraocular pressure and visual acuity follow-up]. Ophthalmologe 2000; 97: 108–12.

Johnson DH, Johnson M. How does nonpenetrating glaucoma surgery work? Aqueous outflow resistance and glaucoma surgery. J Glaucoma 2001; 10: 55–67.

Jonescu-Cuypers C, Jacobi P, Konen W, Krieglstein G. Primary viscocanalostomy versus trabeculectomy in white patients with open-angle glaucoma: A randomized clinical trial. Ophthalmology 2001; 108: 254–8.

Karlen ME, Sanchez E, Schnyder CC, Sickenberg M, Mermoud A. Deep sclerectomy with collagen implant: medium term results. Br J Ophthalmol 1999; 83: 6–11.

Marchini G, Marraffa M, Brunelli C, Morbio R, Bonomi L. Ultrasound biomicroscopy and intraocular-pressure-lowering mechanisms of deep sclerectomy with reticulated hyaluronic acid implant. J Cataract Refract Surg 2001; 27: 507–17.

Massy J, Gruber D, Muraine M, Brasseur G. [Non-penetrating deep sclerectomy in the surgical treatment of chronic open-angle glaucoma. Mid-term results]. J Fr Ophtalmol 1999; 22: 292–8.

Mermoud A. [Deep sclerectomy: surgical technique]. J Fr Ophtalmol 1999; 22: 781–6.

Mermoud A. Sinusotomy and deep sclerectomy. Eye 2000; 14(Pt 3B): 531–5.

Mermoud A, Karlen ME, Schnyder CC et al. Nd:Yag goniopuncture after deep sclerectomy with collagen implant. Ophthalmic Surg Lasers 1999; 30: 120–5.

Mohr A, Rais M, Eckardt C. [Combined cataract-glaucoma surgery with deep sclerectomy. An alternative to gonio-trephination in the intra- and early postoperative phases]. Ophthalmologe 2001; 98: 253–7.

Netland PA. Nonpenetrating glaucoma surgery. Ophthalmology 2001; 108: 416–21.

Roy S, Boldea R, Nguyen C et al. [Analysis of filtration according to implant type after deep sclerectomy in the rabbit]. Klin Monatsbl Augenheilkd 2001; 218: 354–9.

Sanchez E, Schnyder CC, Mermoud A. [Comparative results of deep sclerectomy transformed to trabeculectomy and classical trabeculectomy]. Klin Monatsbl Augenheilkd 1997; 210: 261–4.

Sanchez E, Schnyder CC, Sickenberg M et al. Deep sclerectomy: results with and without collagen implant. Int Ophthalmol 1996; 20: 157–62.

Schwenn O, Dick B, Pfeiffer N. [Trabeculotomy, deep sclerectomy and viscocanalostomy. Non-fistulating microsurgical glaucoma operation ab externo]. Ophthalmologe 1998; 95: 835–43.

Shingleton BJ, Kalina PH. Combined phacoemulsification, intraocular lens implantation, and trabeculectomy with a modified scleral tunnel and single-stitch closure. J Cataract Refract Surg 1995; 21: 528–32.

Spaeth GL. The management of patients with conjoint cataract and glaucoma. Ophthalmic Surg 1980; 11: 780–3.

Spinelli D, Curatola MR, Faroni E. Comparison between deep sclerectomy with reticulated hyaluronic acid implant and trabeculectomy in glaucoma surgery. Acta Ophthalmol Scand Suppl 2000; 78: 60–2.

Sunaric-Megevand G, Leuenberger PM. Results of viscocanalostomy for primary open-angle glaucoma. Am J Ophthalmol 2001; 132: 221–4.

Tixier J, Dureau P, Becquet F, Dufier JL. [Deep sclerectomy in congenital glaucoma. Preliminary results]. J Fr Ophtalmol 1999; 22: 545–8.

Unlu K, Aksunger A. Descemet membrane detachment after viscocanalostomy. Am J Ophthalmol 2000; 130: 833–4.

Wild GJ, Kent AR, Peng Q. Dilation of Schlemm's canal in viscocanalostomy: comparison of 2 viscoelastic substances. J Cataract Refract Surg 2001; 27: 1294–7.

10. Alternative techniques to be used with cataract surgery

Howard V Gimbel and Jean E Keamy

INTRODUCTION

The common occurrence of cataracts and glaucoma makes surgery combined to address both problems appealing. With improvements in both cataract surgery and glaucoma surgery, combined procedures have increased in popularity. The main benefit of a combined procedure is that the patient might undergo only one operation. Furthermore, a combined procedure may reduce the risk of postoperative intraocular pressure (IOP) spikes and provide better long-term IOP control than if cataract surgery alone is performed. Trabeculectomy has remained the gold standard for glaucoma surgery. However, this procedure poses many risks that can potentially decrease vision and cause chronic irritation. Some of the risks of trabeculectomy alone include hypotony, blebitis, endophthalmitis, flat anterior chambers, and choroidal detachments. Additional risks with combined trabeculectomy and cataract surgery include hyphema, posterior synechiae, and pupillary capture. In addition, trabeculectomy when combined with cataract surgery is more apt to fail than if done alone.

Because of these issues, alternative techniques which have low risk, are being considered in combination with cataract surgery. Combined procedures could be beneficial, and with alternative glaucoma techniques, the risks may be lower. Endoscopic cyclophotocoagulation (ECP) and trabeculotomy ab externo are two alternative glaucoma procedures that can be combined with cataract surgery. Although they avoid most of the risks of trabeculectomy, they have their own inherent risks and limitations.

ENDOSCOPIC CYCLOPHOTOCOAGULATION

ECP offers the benefits of ciliary process epithelial photocoagulation without the dreaded complications of phthisis, choroidal effusion, hemorrhage, or pain that can occur with transcleral laser cyclodestruction. Combined with cataract surgery, ECP, compared with trabeculectomy, minimizes the risks of hypotony from overfiltration, flat chamber, choroidal effusion, maculopathy, and visual loss and has been shown to provide a measure of IOP control in various studies. Uram (1995) enrolled 20 patients with open angle glaucoma and cataracts for ECP and phacoemulsification with intraocular lens (IOL) implantation. In this study, the IOP fell from a mean of 29.1 to 14.3 mmHg, a decrease of 50.8% over 2 years. The number of glaucoma medications was 1.9 preoperatively and 0.7 postoperatively. None of the patients had visual loss. Ten percent had progression in visual fields at 1 year after surgery, and none of the patients developed phthisis or endophthalmitis. Uram found ECP combined with cataract surgery to be effective and safe.

Gimbel and Chin conducted a pilot study on 21 eyes using ECP combined with cataract surgery. The patients included in the study had open angle glaucoma with coexisting cataract, documented visual field loss, moderate optic nerve damage, and preoperative IOP greater than 17 mmHg. The initial group had a mean preoperative IOP of 19.3 mmHg. At 8 weeks following surgery the mean IOP fell to 14.3 mmHg. The mean IOP decrease at 3 months was 6.2 mmHg. This group also had a 17% reduction in the use of glaucoma medications.

In a retrospective study performed in 1994–1995, Gimbel and Chin looked at 40 eyes undergoing ECP combined with cataract surgery. All

129

patients (mean age 72.8 years) had open angle glaucoma. The mean preoperative IOP was 18.05 mmHg, ranging from 17 to 28 mmHg. An average of 22.3 ciliary processes were treated with an average of 38.8 pulses per eye. All eyes were followed for 6 months. At 6 months postoperatively, the mean IOP decreased 3.7 mmHg. The postoperative IOP ranged from 3 to 27 mmHg with a mean of 15.3 mmHg at 6 months. Preoperatively, the median number of medications was two, and at 6 months the median number of medications was one, a 50% reduction in medications. No phthisis, maculopathy, or visual loss occurred.

This study found that ECP had many benefits, including no additional incisions, no bleeding, good IOP control, and anatomic precision. The laser endoprobe provides highly titratable amounts of laser energy under direct observation of the ciliary body. Unlike transcleral YAG, cyclocryotherapy, or cyclodiathermy, which are disseminated throughout the sclera, and ciliary muscle, ECP is directed at each ciliary process. ECP can be used in controlled or marginally controlled open angle glaucoma, whereas historically cyclodestructive procedures were reserved for end-stage glaucoma. On the other hand, ECP does not work well in poorly controlled endstage glaucoma. In addition, the pressure-lowering effect takes time and results reported here must be compared to the tendency for cataract surgery alone to decrease IOP (Chapter 2).

INSTRUMENTS FOR ENDOSCOPIC CYCLOPHOTOCOAGULATION

ECP is minimally invasive and can easily be combined with cataract surgery. The only additional equipment required is the laser endoscope and the equipment console (Box 10.1). The laser endoprobe has three fiber groupings, image guide, light guide, and laser guide. Two sizes of endoprobes are available for use. The 20-gauge endoprobe with a 70° field of view provides a large and wide view which can be easier for the beginner. It can focus from its tip from 0.5 mm to 15 mm. The 18-gauge endoprobe has a 110° field of view, and a range of

---

Box 10.1 Surgical instruments

Endoscopic cyclophotocoagulation equipment
Endolaser probe and console
Trabeculotomy ab externo equipment
Diamond knife
Fukaska probe
Fukaska forceps
OPD-SG Posner diagnosis and surgical prism
Viscoelastic

---

focus from 1 mm to 30 mm. The smaller gauge endoprobe allows one to be in focus right on top of the tissue. The laser endoscope attaches to the console, which includes a light source, a video camera, a video monitor, a video recorder, a semiconductor diode laser at 810 nm, and fluorescein imaging ability. With the console placed next to the surgery table, the surgeon views the operating field by looking at the monitor and not through the microscope.

ENDOSCOPIC CYCLOPHOTOCOAGULATION: TECHNIQUE

The ciliary processes can easily be approached from an anterior segment incision. This incision can be either limbal, scleral or in clear cornea, depending on the preference of the cataract surgeon. Phacoemulsification and IOL insertion is first performed, followed by ECP.

For ECP, additional viscoelastic is placed over the capsular bag and posterior to the iris in the quadrant opposite to the incision. The viscoelastic material in the sulcus enhances visualization of the ciliary process and creates ample room for manipulation of the probe. This 'over the bag' technique is also used for phakic and pseudophakic eyes. Alternatively, Uram and others use a 'through the bag' technique. First the capsular bag is filled with sodium hyaluronate. The laser endoprobe is then inserted into the bag and the ciliary processes are visualized through the bag's equator. Following ECP, the intraocular lens is introduced. In both techniques, the laser energy is delivered in a very controlled manner. The goal is to produce whitening of ciliary processes and tissue shrinkage; 180° or more of the circumference of the ciliary body can be treated. One should avoid gas bubble formation, pigment dispersion and a 'popping' sound, all of which indicate tissue disruption and too high of an energy level. One should also avoid photocoagulation of nonciliary process tissue. Periodically, the surgeon should look through the operating microscope to make sure the probe is in the anatomically correct position, and there is no downward, upward, or sideways pressure on the wound edges.

Technically speaking, ECP is quite a safe procedure. Different skills are required because the surgeon directs and evaluates the treatment by looking at a monitor rather than looking through the microscope. Because this takes eye/hand coordination of a different nature than is typically required in ocular surgery, there is a learning curve. If there are any burrs or rough places on the endoscopic probe and care is not taken when manipulating or removing the probe, the iris can be snagged and torn. The ciliary processes are quite easy to identify, but theoretically the laser energy could be applied to the wrong tissue if visualization is poor and the position of the target is uncertain.

One would think that this much destruction of tissue would result in an inflammatory response; however, clinical experience does not consistently show this. Some investigations have reported an increase in cells and flare and cystoid macular edema.

There is a theoretical concern that with the destruction of more than half of the ciliary processes, the eye may suffer from decreased aqueous production. Clinical results to date indicate that there is enough aqueous produced by the remaining ciliary processes. There may be recovery of some of the treated processes because ocular hypotony or degeneration is not observed.

Longer-term follow-up is necessary to fully determine the place of this technique in the arsenal of glaucoma surgery, particularly glaucoma surgery combined with cataract surgery.

TRABECULOTOMY AB EXTERNO

Trabeculotomy has been used for several years to reduce IOP in glaucoma.

In 1960, Smith used a nylon suture threaded into Schlemm's canal to rupture the trabecular meshwork. He reported normalization of IOP in 50% of eyes. Two years later, Allen and Burian named the procedure trabeculotomy ab externo. Harms and Dannhein in 1970 ruptured the trabecular meshwork with a steel wire via a scleral approach. In 1974, Maselli et al used diathermotrabeculotomy to break the trabecular meshwork and Schlemm's canal. However, Luntz and Livingston reported in 1977 a 30% long-term failure rate with trabeculotomy. In 1988, Fukasaku used new forceps and new probes without handles to perform trabeculotomy combined with phacoemulsification.

Gimbel and Meyer in 1995 conducted a prospective, randomized clinical trial on combined trabeculotomy ab externo and phacoemulsification with IOL implantation versus phacoemulsification and IOL implantation in 106 subjects. Glaucoma medications and IOP were evaluated at 3, 6, 12, and 24 months. The preoperative mean IOP in the combined trabeculotomy ab externo and phacoemulsification group was 20.3 mmHg and fell to 14.2 mmHg by 24 months. There was a mean reduction in the IOP of 6.1 mmHg in the combined group and of 3.1 mmHg in the noncombined group at 24 months. There was no increase in medications in either group. The combined group had two complications (2/50), a small tear in Descmet's membrane and a postoperative microhyphema. No surgical complications were noted in the noncombined group.

Trabeculotomy ab externo creates a patent fistula between the aqueous and Schlemm's canal. Because the cataract incision is tightly closed and no filtering bleb is developed, this procedure minimizes the risk of a flat anterior chamber. In the Gimbel and Meyers study, the dreaded complications of choroidal effusion, blebitis, endophthalmitis, flat anterior chambers, maculopathy, and hypotony did not occur. This study showed that phacoemulsification with trabeculotomy ab externo lowers IOP for at least 2 years after surgery without the complications seen with trabeculectomy.

TRABECULOTOMY AB EXTERNO: TECHNIQUE

The Gimbel technique is a modification of the Fukasaku technique. A 7–8-mm limbal-based conjunctival flap is dissected. A straight or frown scleral incision 3–6 mm in length is made 2 mm from the limbus at 12 o'clock. With a diamond knife, the scleral incision is dissected anteriorly at three-fifths scleral thickness (Figure 10.1). This forms a deep

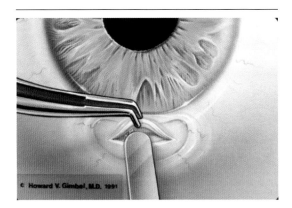

Figure 10.1 Scleral flap incision dissected with a crescent diamond knife.

scleral tunnel over Schlemm's canal. The incision is not continued into the anterior chamber.

Before entering Schlemm's canal, the surgeon must properly identify it. Usually the thin sclera overlying the canal has a darker color which is located just anterior to the scleral spur. With a diamond knife, a radial incision enters the roof of the canal (Figure 10.2). The single staple-like Fukasaku probe is then nudged into the canal, first nasally then temporally. Guiding the tip of the probe against the scleral side of Schlemm's canal enables the probe to enter more easily with less risk of exiting prematurely into the anterior chamber; however, some resistance is normally encountered (Figure 10.3). In its proper position, the probe will be stable and perpendicular to the globe. The OPD-SG Posner diagnostic and surgical prism on a handle may be used to verify the position of the probe (Figure 10.4). The proper position is signaled by a lacy veil overlying a metallic reflex. The view can be improved by deepening the anterior chamber with balanced salt solution or viscoelastic through a medial or lateral paracentesis. If the probe is placed too posteriorly and behind the scleral spur, when it is then rotated into the anterior chamber, a hyphema could occur.

The Fukasaku forceps with a single and a double groove allow the probe crossbar to be held firmly with the single groove of one forceps and rotated with the double groove of the other. Before rota-

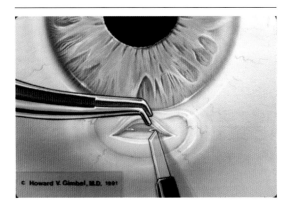

Figure 10.2 Longitudinal incision of the roof of Schlemm's canal.

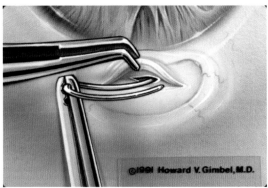

Figure 10.3 Threading the trabeculotomy probe into Schlemm's canal.

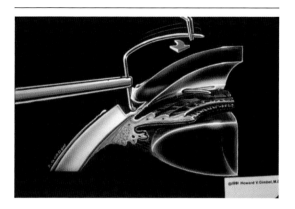

Figure 10.4 Gonioscopic view confirming proper placement of the trabeculotomy probe.

tion, one should puncture the trabecular meshwork with the tip of the probe so as not to detach Descemet's membrane. The vertical cross bar is held firmly and then the external arm of the probe rotates 90° (Figures 10.5 and 10.6). This breaks the trabecular meshwork (Figures 10.7 and 10.8). Keeping slight downward pressure prevents the surgeon from stripping Descemet's membrane (Figure 10.9). One might see heme in the anterior chamber. This heme is due to reflux through the aqueous veins; it usually stops when the IOP is increased with the injection of BSS or viscoelastic through the paracentesis. The probe is then removed and the procedure is repeated in the

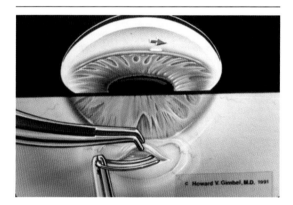

Figure 10.5 Using forceps and trabeculotomy probe to initiate trabeculotomy.

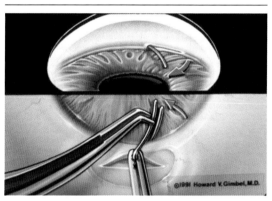

Figure 10.7 Probe is rotated 90° toward the pupil center to complete trabeculotomy.

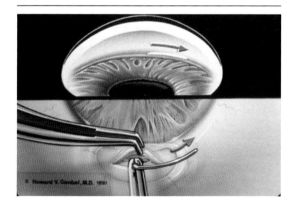

Figure 10.6 Threading the trabeculotomy probe into Schlemm's canal viewed with the aid of goniolens.

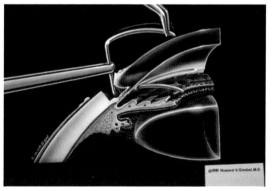

Figure 10.8 Cross-sectional view demonstrating trabeculotomy procedure.

opposite direction. Once the trabeculotomy is completed, a keratome enters the anterior chamber
through the same scleral tunnel incision, and then
a continuous capsulorhexis is made. The lens is
phacoemulsified, and the IOL is inserted.

If the radial incision over Schlemm's canal is
very small, it may be self-sealing along with the
scleral tunnel, and may not require a suture. If it is
not self-sealing, a cross-stitch of 10-0 nylon or
polypropylene suture closes the incision (Figure
10.10). A single 10-0 Vicryl suture or cautery is
used to approximate the overlying conjunctiva.

Postoperatively, the patients are placed on a
nonsteroidal anti-inflammatory agent, a topical
antibiotic, and decreasing glaucoma medications.
Glaucoma medications are not reduced until at
least 1 month after surgery and then only one at a
time.

Three months postoperatively, the patency of
the fistula is assessed. On gonioscopy, a break in the
trabecular meshwork is identified by the loss of pigment. If it is difficult to see the break in the trabecular meshwork to confirm the patency of the
fistula, ask the patient to look down to increase the
pressure on the sclera by the lens. This will increase
the episcleral venous pressure causing the trabeculotomy fistula to fill with blood, which then may
enter the anterior chamber and confirm the
patency of the fistula.

INTRAOPERATIVE COMPLICATIONS

The greatest challenge is to find and thread the
probe into Schlemm's canal. This requires excellent
knowledge of the the anatomy of the surgical limbus and Schlemm's canal. Gaining this knowledge
through the use of fluorescein injected into
cadaver eyes may familiarize the beginner surgeon
with the canal's anatomy. One must always
remember that the distance between Schlemm's
canal and the limbus varies from individual to
individual. A technique during surgery which may
make the canal more visible is to temporarily
increase the episcleral venous pressure by com-
pressing the jugular vein on the same side as the
surgical eye. If one dissects and inserts the probe
too far posteriorly, not inside the canal, rotating
the probe can tear the iris root and cause a
hyphema. Gonioscopy will help verify whether one
is in the canal or not; however, for the transition
surgeon, this may be difficult. If bleeding occurs,
irrigation should be used until it stops to help
minimize residual blood in the anterior chamber.
Unfortunately, the chance to complete the trabeculotomy may be lost at this point, and the
cataract surgery has to be delayed a few minutes
until visualization is restored. A future surgery
may be required for glaucoma control.

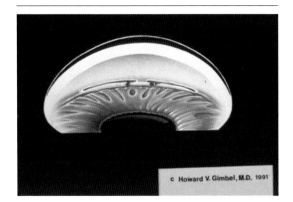

Figure 10.9 Cross-sectional view demonstrating completion of trabeculotomy.

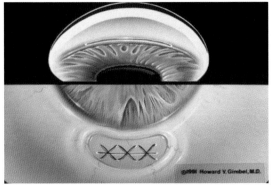

Figure 10.10 Closure of scleral tunnel with running cross-stitch suture.

CONCLUSION

ECP and trabeculotomy have not been widely embraced by North American surgeons, where trabeculectomy has remained the standard practice. Perhaps, the negative results of transcleral cyclophotocoagulation have made many surgeons hesitant to perform ECP. These are, however, not the same procedure. Unlike transcleral cyclophotocoagulation, ECP does not destroy the ciliary body; ECP focuses on destroying just the ciliary process epithelium, posing different but fewer risks than transcleral cyclophotocoagulation. For this reason, ECP warrants further consideration.

Trabeculotomy also deserves further study. With previous technology and instrumentation, trabeculotomy did not achieve great success. Today with new techniques and instruments, trabeculotomy is being done routinely by some surgeons outside North America, such as in Japan and Germany.

FURTHER READING

Allen L, Burian HM. Trabeculotomy ab externo; a new glaucoma operation: technique and results of experimental surgery. Am J Ophthalmol 1962; 53: 9–26.

Birge HL. Glaucoma and cataract surgically cured by single operation. Trans Am Ophthalmol Soc 1952; 50: 241–63.

Chihara E, Nishida A, Kodo M et al. Trabeculotomy ab externo: an alternative treatment in adult patients with primary open angle glaucoma. Ophthalmic Surg 1993; 24: 735–9.

Gimbel HV, Meyer D. Small incision trabeculotomy combined with phacoemulsification and intraocular lens implantation. J Cataract Refract Surg 1993; 19: 92–6.

Gimbel HV, Meyer D, DeBroff B, Roux C, Ferensowicz M. Intraocular pressure response to combined phacoemulsification and trabeculotomy ab externo versus phacoemulsification alone in primary open-angle glaucoma. J Cataract Refract Surg 1995; 21: 653–60.

Greve EL, Wagemans MJ. The combined or triple procedure: extracapsular cataract extraction and filtering surgery in patients with coexisting open angle glaucoma or ocular hypertension and cataract. In: Greve EL, ed. Surgical Management of Coexisting Glaucoma and Cataract. Amsterdam: Kugler Publications, 1987; 69–74.

Fukasaku H, Poliak CR. Trabeculotomy versus trabeculectomy. Trans-Pacific Acad Ophthalmology 1989; May–June: 879–91.

Harms H, Dannheim R. Epicritical consideration of 300 cases of trabeculotomy 'ab externo'. Trans Ophthalmol Soc UK 1969; 89: 491–9.

Harms H, Dannhein R. Trabeculotomy – results and problems. Adv Ophthalmol 1970; 22: 121–31.

Heston JP, Gimbel HV, Crichton AC. The role of small incision cataract surgery in combined cataract and glaucoma surgery. Curr Opin Ophthalmol 1996; 7: 2–10.

Kinoshita A. Comparative study between trabeculectomy and trabeculotomy in fellow eyes. Folia Ophthalmol Jpn 1991; 42: 937–41.

Luntz MH. The advantages of trabeculotomy over goniotomy. J Pediatr Ophthalmol Strabismus 1984; 2: 150.

Luntz MH, Livingston DG. Trabeculotomy ab externo and trabeculectomy in congential and adult-onset glaucoma. Am J Ophthalmol 1977; 83: 174–9.

Mackensen G, Custodis M, Ditzen K. Experiences with trabeculotomy. Can J Ophthalmol 1974; 9: 163–9.

Martin BB. External trabeculotomy in the surgical treatment of congenital glaucoma. Aust N Z J Ophthalmol 1989; 17: 299–301.

Maselli E, Pruneri F, Galantino G et al. Diatermotrabeculotomia ab externo una oculist nuovo tecnica per l'apertura del canale di schlemm. Ann Ottamol Clin 1974; 100: 783–90.

McCartney DL, Memmen JE, Stark WJ et al. The efficacy and safety of combined trabeculectomy, cataract extraction, and intraocular lens implantation. Ophthalmology 1988; 95: 745–62.

McPherson SD Jr. Combined trabeculotomy and cataract extraction. Int Ophthalmol Clin 1981; 21: 87–92.

McPherson SD Jr, McFarland D. External trabeculotomy for developmental glaucoma. Ophthalmology 1980; 87: 302–5.

Murchison JF, Shield MB. An evaluation of three surgical approaches for coexisting cataract and glaucoma. Ophthalmic Surg 1984; 20: 393–8.

Naveh N, Kottass R, Glovinsky J et al. The long term effect of intraocular pressure of a procedure combining trabeculectomy and cataract surgery as compared with trabeculectomy alone. Ophthalmic Surg 1990; 21: 339–45.

Parker JS, Gollamudi S, John G et al. Combined trabeculectomy, cataract extraction, and foldable lens implantation. J Cataract Refract Surg 1992; 18: 582–5.

Rohen JW, Harms H, Barany E. Discussion on new methods of glaucoma surgery. Adv Ophthalmol 1970; 22: 154–8.

Simmons St. Litoff D, Nichols DA et al. Extracapsular cataract implantation combined with trabeculectomy in patients with glaucoma. Am J Ophthalmol 1987; 104: 465–70.

Shields MB. Surgical management of coexisting cataract and glaucoma. In Ritch R, Shields MB, Krupin T, eds. The Glaucomas. St Louis: CV Mosby 1989: 697–706.

Smith R. A new technique for opening the canal of Schlemm; a preliminary report. Br J Ophthalmol 1960; 44: 370–3.

Tanihara H, Negi A, Akimoto M et al. Surgical effects of trabeculotomy ab externo on adult eyes with primary open angle glaucoma and pseudoexfoliation syndrome. Arch Ophthalmol 1993; 111: 1653–61.

Uram M. Endoscopic cyclophotocoagulation in glaucoma management. Curr Opin Ophthalmology 1995; 6: 19–29.

Uram M. Endoscopic fluorescein angiography. Ophthalmic Surg Lasers 1996; 27: 849–55.

Uram M. Endoscopic fluorescein angiography of the ciliary body in glaucoma management. Ophthalmic Surg Lasers 1996; 27: 174–8.

Weldrich A, Manapace R, Radax U et al. Combined small-incision cataract surgery and trabeculectomy-technique and results. Int Ophthalmol 1992; 16: 409–14.

Index

INDEX

pseudoexfoliation glaucoma 73, 84
pseudoexfoliation (PXF) 13, 14
    cataract surgery 16, 18, 19
    and intraocular pressure 15
pseudoexfoliation (PXF) syndrome 13
pseudophakic glaucoma 74, 84
punches 31, 45, 46, 47
pupillary capture 22, 23
pupillary dilation/enlargement 103
    one-site phaco tunnel filtering surgery
        93
    prior to cataract surgery 23, 25–6

releasable sutures 47–8, 50–1, 117
remifentanil 2, 7
renal function 4
respiratory function 5, 7
reticulated hyaluronic acid implants 77
retrobulbar block 7, 8
retrobulbar hemorrhage 7, 116
rocuronium 6

'safety valve' incision 97–9
Sampaolesi line 14
Schlemm's canal
    aqueous drainage 83
    in deep sclerectomy 76, 124, 125
    in trabeculotomy ab externo 132, 134
Schlemm's canal ostia 80
Schwalbe's line 14, 125
scleral ectasia 82
scleral flaps
    combined cataract/NPGS surgery
        122–4
        deeper flap 124–5
    in deep sclerectomy 75–6
    instruments 31
    in trabeculectomy 30, 32–3, 42–5
        closure 47–9
            fixed sutures 47–8
            releasable sutures 47–8, 50–1
        combined with cataract surgery 105
        fashioning 43, 44–5
    in trabeculotomy ab externo 132
    see also conjunctival flaps
scleral tunnel phacoemulsification 115
scleral wound construction 91–2
sclerectomy, deep 71, 72, 75–7
    with collagen implant (DSCI) 71, 77
        in open angle glaucoma 83–4
        vs trabeculectomy 83
    combined with cataract surgery 121, 123
    complications 125–6
    instruments 75
    Nd:YAG goniopuncture after 78
sclero-keratectomy, deep 75–6
sclerostomy 45, 47, 48
    combined with cataract surgery 105
    hyphema 52
sevoflurane 4, 10
sinusotomy 71, 72
sodium nitroprusside see nitroprusside
sphincterotomies 107
staphylomas 65
steroids 5

strabismus 67
Sturge–Weber syndrome 4
subchoroidal space, aqueous drainage
    into 83
subconjunctival blebs 83
succinylcholine 6
suprachoroidal hemorrhage 11
surgical instruments
    cataract surgery 16
    combined cataract surgery
        with drainage device (GDD) 110
        with endoscopic
            cyclophotocoagulation 130
        with NPGS 122
        with trabeculectomy 102
        one-site phaco tunnel filtering
            surgery 91
        trabeculectomy 31
Swan Ganz catheters (SWAN) 3
synechiae
    peripheral anterior 82
    posterior 27

'target' appearance of lens 13
TDM see trabeculo-Descemet's
    membrane
'through the bag' technique 130
timolol 4
trabeculectomy 29–55, 71
    aims 30
    anesthesia 38
    and cataract surgery 29
    combined with cataract surgery 104
        antimetabolites 105
        closure 106
        conjunctival flap choice 104–5
        hazards 106–8
        position 104
        risks 129
    complications 71
    filtration failure 33–5
    indications 29, 102
    and intraocular pressure 29
    intraoperative hazards 51–3
    outflow resistance 33–4
    postoperative care 50–1
    postoperative hazards 53–4
    repeat 30
    risks 53–4, 129
    in secondary glaucoma 29–30
    surgical approach
        antimetabolites 33, 34–6, 38
        conjunctival flap choice 30, 32–3
        drainage bleb 32
        trabeculectomy site 30
    surgical instruments 31
    surgical technique 38–50
        antimetabolite application 39
        conjunctival closure 49–50
        conjunctival dissection 39
        paracentesis 39, 40–1, 52
        peripheral iridectomy 46–7, 53
        scleral flap 30, 32–3, 42–5
            closure 47–9, 50–1
        sclerostomy 45, 47, 48, 52
        traction suture 38, 39

Watson-style 45
    without phacoemulsification
        advantages 30
        in cataract surgery, complicated 30
        and conjunctival scarring 29, 34–5
trabeculectomy block 45, 46
trabeculo-Descemet's membrane 71
    flow through in NPGS 82
    histology 72
    perforation after NPGS 78–80, 81–2
    perforation management 79–80
trabeculoplasty see argon laser
    trabeculoplasty
trabeculotomies 27
trabeculotomy ab externo 71, 72
    cataract surgery with 131–4
        advantages 131–2
        complications 134–5
        postoperative care 134
        surgical technique 132–4
trabeculotomy probe 132
traction sutures
    in drainage implant placement 59, 61
    in trabeculectomy 38, 39
transesophageal probes 1, 3
trigeminal–vagal (oculocardiac) reflex
    10
tropicamide (Mydriacyl) 16, 103

ultrasound biomicroscopy (UBM) 83
upper respiratory infections 4, 11
uveitis
    and combined cataract/GDD surgery
        118–19
    glaucoma after 74

van Lint block 8, 10
vecuronium 6
Versed (midazolam) 7, 10, 103
viscocanalostomy 71–2, 78
    combined with cataract surgery 121
    complications 125
    instruments 75
viscoelastic agents 19
    in cataract surgery 16, 18, 22
        dispersive 20
        'over the bag' technique 130
    in TDM perforation 80
    in trabeculectomy 31, 53
vitreous loss 19
vitreous presentation 53

Watson-style trabeculectomy 45
wet-field cautery 80
wound leak
    after cataract/GDD surgery 117
    after NPGS 80

xylocaine topical jelly 16

Zofran (ondansetron) 11
zonular instability/weakness 107–8
    in cataract surgery 18, 19
    evaluation 14
    in phacodonesis 22
        support 22

140

Management of Cataracts and Glaucoma